CHRONICALLY ILL

Patients

ANGER AND DEPRESSION

SHAZIA YUSUF

TABLE OF CONTENT

LIST OF TABLES

LIST OF FIGURES

LIST OF APPENDICES

ABSTRACT

Present study was conducted to explore the commonly reported psychological issues among chronically ill patients and to explore the risk and protective factors with regard to their impact on well-being and quality of life of patients. Cancer, cardiac and diabetic patients (as per WHO, these three are among top ten causes of deaths in year 2010, NVSS, 2013) were taken from Oncology, General medicine and Cardiology department of Pakistan Institute of Medical Sciences Islamabad (PIMS)). The objectives and hypotheses were formulated within the theoretical framework of Diathesis stress model, self -determination theory and disability stress coping strategy theory.

The research was completed in two parts. Part- I of the study comprised of three phases. Phase I dealt with the Identification of psychological issues, risk and protective factors (through focus groups and in-depth interviews) by using multi-informant approach (patients, caregivers, doctors, nurses and para-medics). Data was analyzed through content analysis. Inter-rater reliability was established for both focus group discussion (Krippendorff's alpha = .89) and interviews (Krippendorff's alpha = .83). The findings of this phase suggested psychological issues faced by patients. Through committee approach the indicators of these issues were labeled in two major groups i.e., depression and anger, whereas the other indicators were grouped as social support and coping strategies (which can be figured out as a risk and protective factor). Beck Depression Inventory (Khan, 1996) was used to assess the depression among patients, Social Support Scale (Malik, 2002) for the assessment of social support, Coping Strategies Questionnaire (Kausar & Munir, 2004) for the assessment of coping strategies, WHO Quality of Life Questionnaire (Khalid & Kausar, 2006) for the assessment of quality of life, Psychological wellbeing scale (Ansari, 2010) was used for the assessment of psychological well-being and for the assessment of anger an indigenous scale was developed. Phase – II dealt with the development of the scale to measure the anger among chronically ill patients. This phase was divided into three steps i.e., review of literature and previous scales, item pool generation and the Exploratory Factor Analysis (KMO = .71). Three factors emerged i.e., state anger (11 items, anger control-in (8 items) and anger control – out (6 items). The content validity was established. In Phase-III of present research, the psychometric properties of all the instruments were established on a sample of 300 patients were taken from PIMS and it was found that scale have sound psychometric properties i.e., alpha coefficients, item total correlations and inter-scale correlations.

Part II of the study was conducted on a sample of 500 chronically ill patients. The results revealed that there is a significant negative relationship between depression, state anger, anger control-in and anger control-out with psychological well-being and quality of life. Multiple regression revealed predictive role of depression, state anger, anger control-in and anger control-out for the psychological well-being ((depression predicting environmental mastery (β = -.46, p = .000) and state anger predicting environmental mastery (β =.15, p = .000), (prediction of autonomy from depression (β = .37, p = .000) and from anger control-in (β =-.14, p = .000), (prediction of personal growth from depression (β = -.46, p = .000) and from state anger (β =.13, p = .003), (prediction of positive relations from depression (β = .03, p = .000) and from anger control-in (β =-.09, p = .02), depression predicting purpose in life ((β = -.45, p = .000), prediction of self-acceptance from depression (β = -.39, p = .000) and anger control-in (β =.13, p = .003)) and quality of life (predicting physical functioning from state control-out (β = -.21, p = .000), (predicting psychological functioning from state anger (β = -.31, p = .000), from anger control-in (β = -.10, p = .01) and from anger control-out (β = .35, p = .000), prediction of social relations from depression (β = .12, p = .01), from state anger (β = -.26, p = .000) and from anger control-in (β = -.16, p = .000), and predicting environment from state anger (β = -.36, p = .000), from anger control-in (β = -.15, p = .000) and from anger control-out (β = .33, p = .000) among chronically ill patients. To find out the moderating role of coping strategies and social support analysis was computed and results supported the hypotheses that coping strategies i.e., social support (tangible support, social network support) significantly play the moderating role in relationship between depression and psychological well- being (self - acceptance, positive relationship with other and autonomy), whereas esteem support acted as moderator between relationship of state anger and psychological well -being (environmental mastery, personal growth). MANOVA was computed on the demographic variables which were further explored with the ANOVA analysis. The significant multivariate main effect of education and marital status, education with age was followed by univariate analyses of variance, which revealed significant differences in depression, informational support, social network support, environmental mastery, self-acceptance, autonomy, purpose in life and personal growth. Tangible support (female M = 17.18, SD = 3.17, Males M = 16.42, SD = 15.29), environmental mastery (female M = 33.01, SD = 13.46, Males M = 27.38, SD = 4.60), positive relations with others (female M = 34.76, SD = 10.50, Males M = 29.92, SD = 11.93) and personal growth (females = 32.06, SD = 10.49, Males M = 28.27, SD = 10.59) is significantly high among female patients as compared to males. Depression is significantly high among those patients who are from nuclear family system (Nuclear M = 16.74, SD = 15.36, Joint M= 13.51, SD = 11.23) whereas environmental mastery (Nuclear M = 29.47, SD = 14.39, Joint M = 34.29, SD = 13.40), positive relations with others (Nuclear M = 32.02, SD = 11.39, Joint M= 35.51, SD = 10.38) and personal growth (Nuclear M = 29.09, SD = 10.90, Joint M = 32.44, SD = 10.41) is high among those patients who are from joint family system. Concluding the present study, depression and anger were figured out as commonly reported psychological issues. Avoidance focused and active distractive coping strategies play risk factor for psychological well-being and quality of life, whereas active focused and religious focused coping strategies along with high level of social support play significant role as protective factors. The present study has important implications in devising a proper treatment plan for chronically ill patients.

Chapter- I

INTRODUCTION

Health is not only linked with physical aspect of one's life but also with the other aspects of his or her life. World Health Organization (WHO) in 1948 has mentioned that absence of disease is not ensuring that someone is healthy, health is beyond this state. It is a condition in which all the domains i.e., physical, mental, emotional and social of one's life, are in harmonious relationship with one another (WHO, 2006). Suffering from chronic disease is uncontrollable event of one's life, it has always weakened down the capabilities of the person and also adversely affected his or her mental well-being.

Chronic diseases always add up to the suffering of one's life. Large number of people from the whole population is targeted by number of diseases and mortality rates are rising increasingly. According to WHO (2012), these (chronic diseases or illnesses) have two important characteristics linked with them. One is duration (long) and the other one is progression which is generally low in them. Heart diseases, cancer, diabetes, respiratory diseases etc are so far the principal cause of disease. It basically stands for sixty-three percent of all deaths. In 2008, large numbers of deaths were caused by chronic illnesses, comprised of approximately thirty-six million people. Many were under 60 years (nine million), whereas ninety percent were from lower socio-economic status (WHO, 2012).

Chronic diseases also accompany psychological disorders along with them (Gregurek, Braš, Đor, Ratković, & Brajković, 2010). There are certain psychological issues which are associated with certain diseases i.e., as certain psychological issues are associated with cancer (Bodurka-Bevers et al., 2000; Katon & Sullivan, 1990; Wells, Golding, & Burnam, 1988), certain with cardiac diseases (Friedman, 2000; Katon & Sullivan, 1990) and certain with diabetes (Anderson, Freedland, Clouse, & Lustman, 2001; Lustman, Clouse, Griffith, Carney, & Freedland, 1997).

Psychological problems accompanying the chronic illnesses can take any form (Verhaak, Heijmans, Peters, & Rijken, 2005). The increasing numbers of chronically ill patients face many difficulties in dealing with their painful condition, the issue is not only linked with the medical care but also linked with meeting their needs for effective clinical management, psychological support and information. Heath care programs are developed by the government to deal with all chronic illness related issues (Wagner et al., 2014). According to the reports and statistics, non-communicable diseases are putting a lot of load as compared to the communicable diseases in terms of the mortality, particularly in lower socio economic status countries where reasons for the 80% death are these diseases (WHO, 2013).

According to the World Federation for Mental Health (WFMH) there is a need for continued and integrated care for chronically diseased patients. There is a very close relationship between the chronic illnesses and the psychological problems. The rate of psychological illnesses increased dramatically in the last two decades. People with the chronic illnesses have elevated level of depression, anxiety and many other psychological problems (WFMH, 2010).

There are many factors associated with the chronic illness like stress, coping and well-being relation. The effects of stress on perception of quality of life and patient's satisfaction with their life, is linked with disease status. Stress may be caused by daily hassles in case of healthy people, and life threatening events in the case of chronically ill people. The psychosocial variables like, personal control, future orientation, optimism and family relations moderate the effect of stress, through the appraisal of the situations. When a person learns that he has developed a life threatening and long lasting illness, he may become dejected and may think that his or her life is over, or he/she may remain optimistic and arguing that new advancement in medicine, he/she will be able to conquer his/her disease (Dubey, 2012).

There are many factors which aggravate the level of psychological issues whereas, there are certain factors which are protective factors, which help in restoring the health and have positive impact on both well-being and quality of life of patients. Bio-psycho-social (behavioral, psychological, and social) risk factors involved in the development and advancement of chronic diseases. Schwartz (as cited in Dubey, 2012) explained that there are many factors which can casue illnesses and these have multiple effects. The important feature of this model is that it not only explains the treatment methods but also suggests different methods to maintain a healthy condition of an individual (Dubey, 2012). The behavioral factors include the risk factors like improper and imbalanced diet, excessive drinking behavior, shared brushes and needles, no going exercise, smoking etc. The Psychological risk factors include aggression and depression whereas societal factors include low education, unclear and uncertain job status etc. These are certain factors contribute as risk in developing negative psychological outcomes of these chronic diseases (Schneiderman, 2004). Positive psychological well-being is related with the cardiac health of the individual (Boehm, Peterso, Kivmaki, & Kubzansky, 2011). Emotional disorders like depression and anxiety are linked with adverse effects on patient's wellbeing and quality of life (Edward, 2013).

The existing literature provide strong evidences regarding psychological issues of chronically ill patients but no comprehensive comparative study is available up to researcher's knowledge that may encompass multiple psychological indicators that can play role as risk factor to patients well-being and quality of life. Further, with the emergence of positive psychology, the research has also focused on positive factors that can play role as protective factors to enhance one's functioning in life. So keeping in view the need, present study was designed to explore psychological issues of chronically ill patients. It has been also focused to identify certain factors that can play significant role in enhancing or deteriorating the mental health, which is directly linked with one's physical health.

Chronic Diseases and Psychological Issues

According to 2010 report, at birth of an individual the expected life years are approximately 78.7 years. Furthermore, the report indicated that 15 leading causes of death in year 2010, were diseases of heart, malignant neoplasms (cancer), mellitus (diabetes) chronic lower respiratory, cerebrovascular diseases (stroke), accidents etc. (NVSS, 2013). It has been reported that among US adults about approximately half of them have at least one of the chronic disease like diabetes, cancer, coronary heart disease, current asthma etc. (Ward, Schiller, & Goodman, 2014). Chronic illnesses contributed in the high mortality and disability rate. In the country like Pakistan about 42 percent of the deaths are because of chronic diseases. The burdens of chronic illnesses like cancer in which person not only have physiological constraints with him but also the deterioration of quality of life and work performance or sometimes discontinuation of the job (Short, Vasey, & Bellue, 2008).

In one of the report it is estimated that approximately around 3.87 million will die because of non communicative diseases i.e., cancers, chronic respiratory and cardiovascular diseases. It was also highlighted that financial constraints are associated with the non communicable diseases (Jafar et al., 2013).

All chronic diseases have some common characteristics which are given below.

1. Chronic conditions may range from mild to severe life threatening disorders. It may be as mild as the hearing loss and as severe as the stroke. The onset of the chronic illness is very slow but it is progressive in nature.

2. Contrasting with the acute diseases that are caused by some virus, chronic diseases are caused by multiple factors; behavior and life style of the person plays very important or vital role. As in the case of heart diseases the low physical activity, unhealthy dietary habits and stress.

3. Chronic diseases are manageable with the change in life style and with the help of medication, condition can be controlled. Health conditions vary from disease to disease (Ghosh, 2015).

In WHO report it was mentioned that out of ten causes of death, the top seven were chronic diseases. Heart diseases and cancer contributed in nearly forty-eight percent of all deaths. Furthermore, this report illustrate that many deaths are caused because of diabetes. These three chronic diseases were enlisted as top leading cause or reason behind large number of deaths (CDC, 2013).

Cardiovascular diseases. Round the globe it is quite evident that cardiovascular diseases (CVDs) are one of the main prominent causes of death. Annually many people die because of it as compared to any other cause. In 2008 approximately 17.3 million people died because of cardiovascular diseases, which represent 30% of deaths (globally). 6.2 million died because of stroke and 7.3 million died because of CVDs (WHO, 2011).

According to the updated fact sheet of World Health Organization (WHO), the world wide leading cause of death is CVDs. Many people die annually because of CVDs. According to WHO in Pakistan fifty percent of the deaths are because of Non-Communicable diseases and CVDs causes for nineteen percent of the deaths (WHO, 2014). Furthermore, it has been reported that in lower and middle income countries, over three quarters deaths are because of CVD. People living in lower and middle income countries do not have facilities to avail the primary health care facilities so most of the time there is a late detection and survival is difficult, that's why the death rates from heart diseases are very high (WHO, 2017). Cardiovascular diseases are the main reason for eighty percent deaths in under developed countries. Individuals from the under developed countries are more vulnerable to the hazardous factors which may lead them to develop cardiovascular diseases and other NCDs. Basically they don't have opportunity to have get effective and up to date health facilities (WHO, 2011). Approximately 800,000 deaths in US are because of cardiovascular diseases and in every 40 second an average person dies because of it. According to one report by 2030 the estimated cost for the cardiovascular disease will be $1,044 billion (Benjamin et al., 2017).

The heart attacks and strokes are considered as critical incidences in someone's life and are because of blockage inside the blood vessels that's why the supply of the blood gets disturbed or disrupted. This will then lead to heart attack or stroke. The major and most common reason behind this blockage condition is deposits which are inside the vessels and these are deposits of fats. Blood clotting or blood vessels bleeding in the brain can cause the stroke (WHO, 2012).

There are research evidences that the incidences of psychological changes and cardiovascular changes, explains the complication linked with psycho-somatic and somato-psychic consequences. The factors linked with psychological condition of the person are hostility, depression and anxiety, which affect the heart diseases (from development to prognosis). These are commonly reports by cardiac patients (Ilic & Apostolovic, 2002). Anger is associated with the chronic heart diseases (Davidson & Mostofsy, 2010), furthermore, guilt, sadness, grief and shock considered as a normal reaction at the onset of the disease (heart). These conditions have been commonly reported by these patients (Shapiro, 1996). Higher rates of depression, anxiety and many other psychological problems are common among heart patients (WFMH, 2010). Poor psychological health (e.g., depression) is prospectively associated with adverse cardiac outcomes (Huffman, Legler, & Boehm, 2017). The presence of depression is having adverse effect on prognosis of patients (Barefoot & Schroll, 1996). Cardiac patients and diabetics have adverse quality of life as compared to other patients who were suffering from chronic illness (Chen, Baumgardner, & Rice, 2011).

Cancer. Cancer is the second main reason behind numerous deaths in U.S. The age adjusted cancer death rates are increasing in the US population (Bal & Foerster, 1991). There are many kinds of cancers but the most common include carcinoma, sarcoma, lymphoma and leukemia. There are many other types of cancer, depending on the body part which get affected by the cancer. In Pakistan the registered cases are very few. A big dilemma is that most of the patients die of some chronic illnesses but that never get diagnosed. Karachi Cancer Registry (KCR) was developed for documentation and registration of cancer. It is providing the prevalence of cancer in the country (Bano et al., 2013).

Numerous studies have identified that there are many social and psychological factors play a considerable role in establishing that whether a person can get cancer or not. Many studies have been conducted to explore the role of psychological factors in progression and prognosis of cancer. Furthermore, reviews of many studies summarize that the stressful life events, locus of control, coping strategies, personality factors and social factors play important role in progression of cancer (Dubey, 2012).

Cancer is more closely tied with the life style then to genetics (Lichtenstein et al., 2000). Almost among all type of cancer patients develop some level of distress (psychology) linked with the disease and its treatment (Derogatis, Morrow, & Fetting, 1983). Large number of patients (cancer) experience psychological issue specially the distress in which consultancy specifically psychological consultancy is required. Cancer patients are usually suffering from more psychological problems as compared with the other patients. The diagnosis of having cancer is shocking, heartbreaking and earth shaking for the patients. Lots of problems are linked with the diagnosis of the chronic illness (Heather, Susan, Deanna, & Barbara, 2006; National Cancer Registry, 2003; Senescus, 1963). Adjustment disorders, depression and anxiety are common among patients suffering from cancer (Gregurek et al., 2010). Large number of cancer patients suffers from depression (Asghsremoghadam, 2006). Higher depression and anger was found among younger cancer patients (Hadi, Asadollahi, & Talei, 2009). Major depression is highly and commonly reported by cancer patients (Pasquini & Biondi, 2007).

Depression, adjustment disorders, and anxiety disorders are commonly reported psychiatric disorders among patients suffering from cancer (Gregurek et al., 2010). Patients reported that they have trouble falling to sleep, have no interest in doing something which gives them pleasure, mostly have low mood, depress and hopeless (Que et al., 2013). National Cancer Registry in 2011 has mentioned that the cancer patients suffer from different psychological symptoms i.e., nervousness, they are least concerned about anything, sadness, sleep and eating habits got changed, they are unable to focus on different things and have repetitive thoughts about death (as cited in Yusof, Zakaria, Hashim, & Dasiman, 2016). Patients experience an anger as a response of falling ill (Honorato, Arumusse, Coqueiro, & Citero, 2017). Furthermore, literature has highlighted that as anger is perceived as not socially acceptable in society so mostly it appears in form of depressive symptoms and symptoms of distress (Taylor, Baird, Malone, & McCorkle, 1993). Many psychological factors and social factors like loss of support, absence of current social network, absence of close family ties, it effects the onset and course of of cancer (Dubey, 2012). There are many factors which help in reducing the level of psychological issues among chronically ill patients. Religious coping is significantly negatively associated with the depression (Koenig et al., 1992).

As the mental health issues are very common among cancer patient so there is a need to give them a psychotherapeutic treatment. The effectively of the psychological and psycho-pharmacological treatment should be checked time to time (Gregurek et al., 2010). The concerns which are linked with the cancer are early deaths, dependency on others, issues in social life, physical condition of the person gets affected and employment. Because of the treatment the person's reproductive capacity gets affected, and concerns about future may cause distress among individuals with cancer (Zebrack, 2011). In 20th century (in its second part) psycho-oncology was introduced which is a direct indication of deep interest in the psychological issues of the cancer patients. Psycho-oncology is popular now almost all around the world and departments has been established in US, Western European countries and Canada. The greatest challenge is associated with the understanding of distress linked with distress which may be an expected one or it can be transient, but both require the psychiatric consultancy (Gregurek et al., 2010).

Diabetes. Diabetes mellitus is linked with the hyperglycemia and is common metabolic disorder. It's basically associated with the condition in which the person has an excessive glucose level in his or her blood stream (Carver & Abrahamsom, 2009). It appears in a reaction of defect in insulin action or secretion or both (Taylor, 2009). It has been explained by American Diabetes Association (ADA) that there are two major categories of diabetes are that 1) type 1 and type 2 (as cited by Javaid, 2014). Those individuals who are suffering from the type 1 diabetes, for their survival they are dependent on insulin (Carver & Abrahamsom, 2009; CDC, 2007). According to the reports of ADA, these patients have indicated that 90 to 95% of the diabetic cases are having diagnosis of type 2 diabetes (as cited by Javaid, 2014). Type 2 is described as a condition in which the body is unable to utilize the insulin properly and this condition is because of their insulin resistance. In start of this issue, pancreas is able to properly counterbalance the resistance by enhancing insulin. But with the passage of time, the cells in the pancreas fail to maintain the insulin secretion and as it's not up to the normal level, thus it is leading to the development diabetes mellitus (ADA, 2013).

It has been reported that worldwide about three hundred and forty-six million people are having diabetes. The most horrifying situation is that they do not have knowledge about their disease and its current status or condition (UN News Centre, 2012). In a survey, it has been concluded that in Pakistan, prevalence of diabetes is quite alarming as among the males its 5.1% whereas 6.8% in females, living in urban areas (Aziz, Noorulain, Zaidi, Hossain, & Siddiqui, 2009).

Pakistan is having many diabetic patients whose condition is very alarming and it is ranked as having a seventh position for the prevalence and disease burden of diabetes mellitus. As the conditions are deteriorating day by day and if the condition persists then Pakistan will move from seventh to fourth position for diabetes mellitus prevalence. At present, in Pakistan about 12.9 million individuals are having diabetes (DIP, 2013).

Diabetes requires a complex self-management and medical treatment. There are certain diseases which are not completely curable but are manageable and Diabetes is among one of them. Physiological hardships are something which is unavoidable in nature and psychological issues also accompany the physiological issues, so with deteriorated health they are unable to manage their health. There are certain psychological issues which are very common among the diabetes. Often the healthcare experts, working with diabetic patients fail to recognize the presence of psychological issues among their patients. Unfortunately, approximately two out of three patients, who are suffering from psychological issues, often go undiagnosed (Hermanns, Kulzer, Krichbaum, Kubiak, & Haak, 2006; Pouwer, Beekman, Lubach, & Snoek, 2006).

Patients with chronic conditions often have to adjust their lifestyles and employment. Many patients who are already suffering from chronic illness get diagnosed with depression, hopelessness, mood problems, sometime they have a strong desire to commit suicide and also suffer from other psychological problems (Turner & Brian, 2000). Patients who were suffering from chronic illness (like arthritis, diabetes, cancer, renal disease or dermatological disease patients) were assessed and the results revealed that recently diagnosed patients had a poor mental health as compared to those patients whose illness got diagnosed four months ago. Significant association was found between the physical status of health and the mental health of the patients. Results suggested that adjustment specifically linked with psychological condition, among patients with chronic illnesses is surprisingly effective and basically independent of specific diagnosis (Cassileth et al., 1984).

There are research evidences which clearly indicate the prevalence of psychological problems among chronically ill patients so there is a need to provide a proper psychological treatment to the patients who are also suffering from psychological illnesses (Guthrie, 1996).

Disease related psychological issues are increasing with every passing day. Poorer quality of life for people with this condition is very common observation. It is necessary for the health care personnel that they must be well knowledgeable to identify the problems of the diabetics and should ensure that they are receiving the necessary support (Britneff & Winkley, 2013). Diabetes also increases the risk of depression. Diabetes also increases the risk of depression and develops depression (Anderston, Freedland, Clouse, & Lustman, 2001; Lewko & Misiak, 2015; Mir, Mir, Malik, Quratulain, & Shehzadi, 2015). It is also repeatedly highlighted by the literature that the psychological problems get elevated in patients with diabetes (Lorenz et al., 1996). Anger is also commonly reported by diabetic patients (Solowiejczyk, 2010). Along with anger, depression is also very commonly reported among diabetics (Penckofer, Ferrans, Velsor-Friedrich, & Savoy, 2007). Sleep problems and functional impairments are reported in these patients (Mohamed, Kadir, & Yaacob, 2012). Anger, depression and anxiety are prevalent among diabetics (Muscatello et al., 2017). High levels of depressive symptoms are reported (Vu et al., 2018). Depressive symptoms are high among female diabetic patients (Rezia, Islam, & Islam, 2018). In one study it was concluded that at least one episode of life threatening illness was experienced by almost all males, in which they felt that they will die after a month. On the other hand, the mood disorder and psychiatric distress was also found (Rabkin, Remien, Katoff, & Williams, 1993).

Mental health issues are commonly found among people with diabetes and are also linked with the adverse outcomes. The association between disease (diabetes) control, social factors and mental health means holistic approach is needed. Interventions (psychological) can be used for management of psychological problems (Britneff & Winkley, 2013).

Researches revealed that psychotherapeutic treatment is more effective than antidepressant for the treatment of depression and glycaemic control, especially when combined with self-management education. Psychotherapy, psychological interventions and counseling are the main terms and people referred for psychological therapy may receive different types of verbal therapy (Britneff & Winkley, 2013).

The occurrence of mental illness with chronic illness can deteriorate the self-care and compliance with the treatment, can cause the high mortality rates. Much alarming incidence is that the mental illness is associated with the hindrances in normal functioning of an individual, causing significant impairment in role, causes work loss or work cut down. These (psychological issues) also have worse prognosis for many chronic illnesses like diabetes, HIV/AIDS, cancer, heart disease, stroke and other chronic illnesses. Most of the times patients and their relatives or caregivers are unable to recognize the symptoms or maybe they hesitant or unwilling to seek psychological help. Sometimes the experts those who are providing the psychological consultancy are not properly trained or they are not well equipped with interventions with which they can provide proper help to patients. Financial and other technical constraints are there, with the access and availability of these services (WFMH, 2010).

The multiple issues related to psychological, social and emotional functioning of chronically ill persons have been focused of research in last few decades. Chronic illness is multidimensional in nature, and people who are suffering from it and their caregivers have to do lots of things like looking after and management of treatment, dealing with the symptoms, dealing with crisis, recording time, managing the course of illness, dealing with healthcare experts, normalizing life, maintain self image, keeping a balance in emotional life and dealing with the social isolation (Belgrave, 1998; Lubkin & Larsen, 2013). Chronic illness does not discriminate or differentiate on basis of race, age, socioeconomic status, or gender, there are some children also suffer from the chronic diseases (Newacheck et al., 1998). Among chronically ill patients, depression hostility and anxiety is common (Gregurek et al., 2010).

Theoretical Perspectives

Diathesis-stress model. The diathesis stress model was developed by Holmes and Rahe in 1967 then was expanded by Zubin and Spring then further reformulated by Dr. Robert Liberman and his colleagues (Heller & Gitterman, 2010). It's basically a psychological theory which is dealing with the behavior and mental disorders which are result of biological and genetic vulnerability, and stress linked with the life experiences.

This model explains that sometimes people has the vulnerability or proneness to develop the stress-related diseases. The reason behind the development of the disease may be linked with the either genetic weakness or biomedical imbalance inherently makes them more vulnerable to those diseases. Since, long this model is explaining the development of psychological disorders to the psychologists and other professionals. During the time period of 1960s and 1970s, the concept was used for the explanation for development of psychological disorder (Brannon & Feist, 2009).

According to the model, some individuals have tendency to react abnormally to the stressors (environmental). This tendency of developing disorder is usually thought to be linked with the inheritance, whereas for some experts like Zubin and Spring (as cited in Brannon & Feist, 2009) have also mentioned that person has acquired tendencies as a components of vulnerability (Brannon & Feist, 2009).

Thus, the diathesis stress model assumes that two factors are necessary to for the development of any disease. First, the person should be having a proness or tendency to develop diseases and second is that the person is must going through some sort of stress (Brannon & Feist, 2009). Often there are certain factors which actually play a very important role especially in bringing about that problem (Newton, 2013). However, there are many interceding factors, which are playing the role of shield between the predisposing and precipitating factors. Social support systems can be considered as an important factor, which plays a very important role in preventing a disorder or lessening its severity (Newton, 2013). Considering these buffering positive factors, Diathesis –Stress factors can be prevented with optimal level of functioning and well- being. To understand these positive processes, self-determination theory can be a good explanation.

The frustration – Aggression Hypothesis

It's a common notion that nobody wants to have a health which is detorirated or not complete. History explains that the Dollard et al in 1939 came up with the frustration – aggression hypothesis. As per according to this model, the frustration is caused whenever the goal directed behavior is being blocked by something or someone. This frustration leads to the aggressive behavior in an individual. Everyone wanted to have a complete, good and satisfying life but illness blocks that particular goal of having disease free life. According to Dollard and his colleagues the two main propositions of the aggression are: 1) the occurances of frustration always leads to some form of aggression. 2) The existence of frustration always leads to some form of aggression (DiGiuseppe, & Tafrate, 2007). Having chronic disease make the individual to develop frustration and then this frustration leads to aggression. Aggression is commonly reported by chronically ill patients (Honorato, Arumusse, Coqueiro, & Citero, 2017).

Learned helplessness

Learned helplessness is basically the consequence of exposure of an individual towards an uncontrollable event, as chronic diseases are not in the control of an individual so they feel helpless and consider things as uncontrollable in nature. Personal helplessness causes, when one considers that things are not in his or her control. This feeling of helplessness make individual thinks as worthless and helpless that's why he or she never tries to induce any change in his or her life and losses hopes (Lubkin & Larsen, 2006). The repitive failtures of an individual makes him learn that he is a complete failure no matter whatever the situation is going to be, he will only endup with failure in every area of his life (Dalal, 2015). With the realization of the fact that one is having a chronic illness, is related with the significant impact in one's life. Individuals may suffer or experience the feelings of depression, helplessness, apathy and hopelessness. They feel rejected and dejected (Falvo & Holland, 2017).

Self-determination theory (SDT). Self-determination theory throw a light on all those psychological processes which are promoting the ideal or optimum functioning and health of an individual. SDT postulates three very important and elementary inborn or inbuilt needs (psychological) which includes competence, autonomy and relatedness. These are very basic needs of an individual and which need to be satisfied for the optimum functioning of an individual. These needs are universally present, no matter where ever the individual is living his basic needs are same.

Competence is a need which is linked with the person's ability to get adjusted with the changing environment and atmosphere. It basically helps the individual to adapt to new challenges of life, to arouse his unique talents and does his work in an efficient manner. It helps him or her to meet the demands of the society and show his full potential for any task. But there are certain incidences in one's life which are life changing experiences and totally make a person a change individual. Due to the illnesses the person feels like he doesn't have any control in his life and their sense of autonomy get affected. So with the illness the psychological condition gets effected badly (Lubkin & Larsen, 2013).

Any event in individual's life challenge him to use his or her full potential to come out of that situation. Individual react to any unexpected event by using both (emotional and cognitive) abilities. Chronic illness is a life changing event for some individuals and when there is a chronic illness then definitely it is something which is challenging the individual on both (physical and psychological) levels. When individual encounters any chronic illness or disability then his or her psychological factors effects his response to these events. These illnesses not only effect the functioning and adjustment of an individual but also the course of disease and prognosis (Falvo, 2005). Life style also gets affected. Life style comprises of daily life activities of an individual. These activities are linked with the individual's environment. Activities include preparing food, housekeeping and many other things. The other activities are also included in it like transportation, rest, recreational and many other activities which are important for the life of an individual (Belgrave, 1998).

Health and illness as a continuum. Health psychology is a field of psychology which basically deals with health and illness issues. It takes the health and illness as being a continuum and tries to figure out the ways with which psychological factors effects the heath at all levels and stages. This model emphasized on illness onset which is always linked with psychological problem (e.g., behaviors, stress, and beliefs), help seeking (symptoms perception), illness adaptation (e.g., social support), and illness progression and health outcomes (e.g., quality of life) (Odgen, 2012).

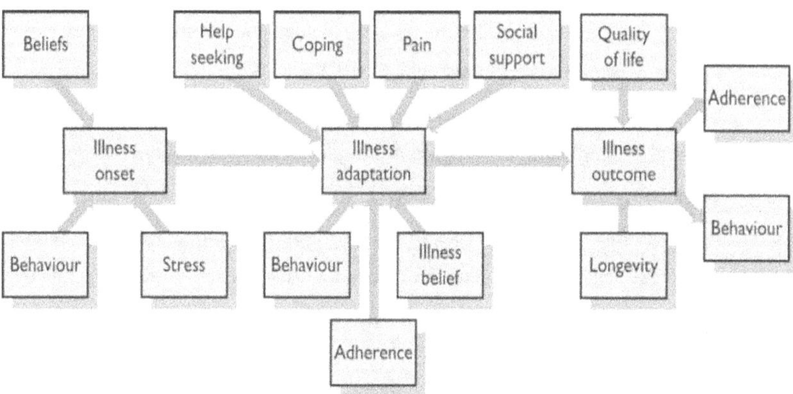

Figure 1. Health and illness as a continuum

Resilience theory. Resilience is a vigorous and active process. It is basically linked with the interaction of protective and risk factors which are very important for the survival of an individual. These factors are directly linked with the normal functioning of the human beings (Fredrikson-Golden, 2007). Risk factors are conceptualized as those events which have adverse effects on adaptive functioning. It has been explained that the approach was shifted to highlight the importance of resilience. And this shift was actually from risk to resilience. Turner (1995) explained that because of the persistent use of strategies for figuring out of risk factors, make people frustrated and made them to look for resilient factors. But the identification of risk factors or in order words the risk focus approach is very effective and helpful in many cases like in the case of infectious diseases. In case of infectious diseases, it can help in identification of risk factors and taking preventive measure for their reduction, whereas in case of more complex diseases the more comprehensive approach is required (Turner, 1995).

The disability-stress-coping model. If the history of Disability-Stress-Coping model (Wallander & Varni, 1989) gets open then it provides the information that it is first initiated by Pless and Pinkerton, Moss, Schaefer and Lazarus and Folkman. It is a model which is linked with the identification of the risk and protective factors which are playing their role in the disease. Wallander and Varni (1989) has explained that there are certain risk factors which are linked with the disease and these factors include 1) parameters which are linked with the disease or disability (for example, medical complications, cognitive impairments, visibility, diagnosis etc.), 2) dependency on others, related to daily living activities and 3) stressors (psychosocial) (stressors like daily life events, disease or disability related problems). These all three major risk factors linked with the diseases or disabilities. Ultimately, this dependency was changed to independence by making minor changes in one's life.

According to Wallander and Varni (1989), protective factors demarcated as having three major categories. 1) interpersonal factors like motivation, character and temper of a person, competence etc. 2) socio-ecological factors which includes social support, family environment specifically the psychological one, family resources available to an individual etc. resources and 3) stress interpretation and dealing factors like coping, cognitive processing, processing of information etc. (Brown, 1999).

Impact of Psychological Issues on Well-Being of Chronically Ill Patients

Numerous approaches describe the dynamics of chronic diseases and their adverse impact on individual's mental health and well being. According to some well renowned psychologists well-being is concept which is linked with good mental and emotional functioning (health), which is contributing in the quality of life of an individual as explained by López and Torres (as cited by Gomez, Gutiérrez, Castellanos, Vergara, & Pradilla, 2010) in various contexts. By keeping in mind all that then the psychological well-being is linked with the approach with which people are looking at their lives and evaluating it (how they are looking at their past, present and future). When one talk about the evaluation of assessment of psychological well-being then it also includes the emotional response of a person towards any event, person etc. it is actually depicting their way of living (Diener, Oishi, & Lucas, 2003).

Psychological well-being was explained as not having any psychological issue (Kasl, Chisholm & Eskenazi, 1981). Furthermore, it is about one's talent to appraise his or her functioning by keeping in mind all the several different but interconnected perspective (like, physical, mental and global) (Schlosser, 1990). In the beginning psychology was majorly focusing on the diagnosis of psychological issues and then doing the treatment of these issues, instead of looking for the strengths which are required for the flourishing of one's sound health. Positive psychology is a branch of psychology which is specifically dealing with the understanding and putting main focus on real happiness, knowledge, insight and psychological well-being (Seligman, 2002).

Everyone wishes to always stay happy in their lives and subjectivity is involved in the experience of feelings of happiness and satisfaction, this experience is called as a psychological well-being (Okun & Stock, 1987). That sort of happiness or subjective happiness is not because of some material gain or something person achieved in his or her life. Psychological well-being is more and more linked with the attitude and approach of a person towards life situations. It's a multi-dimensional concept (Sinha & Verma, 1992).

Psychological well-being is not associated with dearth of distress, tension or pain. It entails about the satisfaction of psychological needs of an individual. Typically, the experts, especially psychologists explained it as recognizing and sharing the value of being together and value this togetherness (Keyes & Lopez, 2002).

Theoretical Perspectives of Psychological Well-Being

Many theories have been proposed to explain the phenomenon of psychological well-being. These theories or paradigms are divided into three categories which include; Need and Goal Satisfaction, process or activity paradigm and genetic and personality predisposition. The need and goal satisfaction paradigm emphasizes on the assumption that in case if the tension is reduced, it makes the person to feel happy. According to this paradigm when the person accomplishes the valued goal he or she attains the psychological well-being. The second paradigm is about the Process or activity paradigm, majorly focuses on the assumption that when the person does the activities which are linked with their intrinsic satisfaction (Sheldon, Rayan, & Reis, 1996). Harlow and Cantor (1996) focused on the importance of the major goals of individuals that when they are engage in the activities linked with the achievement of these goals then they feel very satisfied. The third paradigm is basically Genetic and personality disposition and according to it the personality and genetics intensely effects the psychological well-being of an individual (Synder & Lopez, 2002).

Two domain model. Braddurn (1969) proposed a 2 domain model, he described that the negative and positive effects are two different dimensions; each is playing its role in the psychological well-being of an individual. Negative affect is linked with the unpleasant events and the health complaints (Watson, Clark, & Tellegen, 1988), health complains may include the illness or disease, whereas positive effect is linked with the pleasant events. Many experts not accepted this notion and said that the positive and negative effects are not independent of each other actually they are interlinked with one another. Ferrell (1995) explained that the illness and wellness belongs to one continuum.

Bottom-up model. It explains that the summations of pleasurable and unpleasurable experiences are actually linked with the happiness of an individual. Furthermore, it maintained the view that by simply adding up or summing up the well-being in a particular domain, like family and work, college, people develops well-being (psychological). If summarized this model clearly indicates that the happiness is linked with the particular incidences in one's life (Bryant & Marquez, 1986).

Top-down paradigm. It explains, people have capacity or tendency to construe events of their life as progressive one or deleterious one and this interpretation then leads to the appraisal of gratification of a person in a particular domain. Philosophically this model is linked with the Kantain model (1958). The top down model demonstrates that the main or basic impact on our well-being is because of our personal interpretation of the events rather than neutral or objective evaluation. Most of the researches give importance to the integrated approach (Diener, 2009). Integrated model explains that all the interpretations by individuals will directly influence the psychological well-being of the individual.

Multidimensional paradigm or model. This model is presented by Ryff and Keyes (1995), it's the recent model. They have explained that the well-being (psychological) includes six diverse aspects or categories including: purpose in life, positive relations, self-acceptance, environmental mastery, personal growth, autonomy and personal growth. Ryff and Keyes explained that this paradiym is more comprehensively and meaningfully explains the psychological well-being. According to them it's a multifaceted model. Major components of this model are explained as follow:

Autonomy.   It is basically about one's government or independence which includes qualities like independence and regulation of behavior within. The self-actualizers and the optimally functioning individuals are those who have internal locus of control, in which the individuals do not requires endorsement of others.

Environmental mastery. The individual's ability to create a suitable environment, which is appropriate or suitable for one's physical and ofcourse the mental health. This theory explains the human being's ability to move in his or her life by advancing in life. The theoretical perspectives suggest that environmental mastery is vital ingredient in the positive psychological functioning of an individual.

Personal growth. For proper and complete psychological functioning personal growth is very important. There is a need to actualize one's potential and capabilities to have a personal growth. Openness is the basic and key characteristic for fully functioning person. Such an individual is continually developing excelling in his or her life.

Positive relation with others. Psychological well-being is also linked with establishing warm and trusting relationships with others. The ability to love is viewed as the main and central component of mental health. Self actualizers are considered to have an affectionate feelings and empathetic feelings for everyone. Other development theories also emphasized, on the importance of positive relations with others and taking guidance from others, which is important for one's positive psychological development.

Purpose in life. For a sound mental health, it is important to have some purpose in one's life. The explanation is maturity is also linked with the having some goal of life.

Self acceptance. It is explained as a very important and major feature of sound psychological condition. Its characteristics include maturity, proper and optimum functioning of individuals. Literature and theories of life span supported that for sound mental health, the individual should have his or her acceptance for past life events and above all he should be accepting his or her self. So having a positive attitude towards himself or herself for optimum functioning.

Therefore, well-being is an active and ever changing process, which is continuously changing with every single moment (Ballesteros et al., 2003), according to Skinner it is based on the appraisal of relationships among individuals which are either conditional or functional, and their evaluation about their environment and life conditions (as cited in Ballesteros & Caycedo, 2002), while describing about the role of well-being of an individual it is important to look into different variables and their interaction specially those which are identified by them (individuals). So while making any assessment about chronically ill patients it is important to consider numerous factors which are affecting their lives as for example among cancer patients the diagnosis of disease, stage of disease, treatment and then remission (Goepp & Hammond, 1977) and during the course of the treatment (Novoa-Gómez, Moreno, Garcia, Leguizamón, & Castaño, 2006).

At that time the psychological support is an important factor which can affect patient's adjustment and can play a constructive or destructive role in treatment course. Health status of patients can be determined through quality of life as it's considered as very important or significant element in determining the psychological well-being of a patient. It's true that the way patient perceives the situation it is going to affect his or her health in a same manner (Diener, Oishi, & Lucas, 2003).

Impact of Psychological Issues on Quality of Life of Chronically Ill Patients

The concept of the quality of life gained an abundant importance in the history. Historically the concept of quality of life was primarily used in political science as well as in the social sciences including politicology, anthropology, psychology and sociology. Now recently the term quality of life has been introduced in medicine (Koot & Wallander, 2001). Few decades back the research in the medical area started exploring the concept of quality of life and its significance. In 1970s which was considered as a starting phase of philosophical publications related with the question like what is quality of life and whether it can be measured or not. In 1980s the more and more methodological approaches appeared linked with the instrumentation of quality of life. Since the beginning of the 1990s the third phase of research of quality of life appeared. A fourth phase of suing the quality of life data for quality assurance and health economic evaluation is just beginning. The research in this area is very important and highlighted area "quality of life" resulted in to over 20,000 published articles on the different aspects of it like it's conceptual basis, methodological approaches, assessment and application in different type of studies (Koot & Wallander, 2001).

The literature is abounding with the information related to the effect of chronic illness or disease on quality of life of an individual. The European Organization for Research on Treatment of Cancer explained that quality of life is linked with functional status of a person, symptoms which are related with the cancer and its treatment, expenses, perception of the patient about his or her health and overall quality of life (Aaronson et al., 1993). Chronic illness is often associated with the having depression, anxiety and distresses which considerably increase the risk of death from the chronic illness (Christensen & Lægreid, 2002). Quality of life of chronically ill patient is judged by the disruption in sleep, appetite gets affected and the daily functioning gets affected. In the latter stages and at more chronic stage quality of life is associated with the fact that whether the individual is able to perform independently the daily routine activities like eating, bathing, dressing etc. inability to perform these daily activities independently adversely affect the psychological condition of the person (Ghosh, 2015). Universally, quality of life is assessed based on certain components like performing different daily physical activities, emotionally one is sound, interpersonal relationships, personal control, energy level, social functioning, personal and intellectual growth etc. (Power, Harper, & Bullinger, 1999).

Quality of life is a multifaceted concept which comprehend about both subjective and objective dimensions which include health, housing, food and self-perception etc. (Carpio, Pachecho, Flores, & Canales, 2000; Novoa, Cruz, Rojas, &Wilde, 2003). Diener (cited in Rodriguez-Martin, 1998) has demarcated that the quality of life is a subjective view of a person which is linked with achieving happiness and satisfaction in one's life, subjective view encompasses all the related dimensions (psychological, social, biological, economic) of one's life (Garavito explained, as cited in Gómez, Gutiérrez, Castellanos, Vergara, & Pradilla, 2010).

The World Health Organization has combined their efforts to squeeze the complexity and explain it one terminology which is "Quality of Life", they have explained it as a insight of a person in his or her own existence, in accordance to their cultural and value system in which they are living in particular relation to their expectations, norms and concerns etc. it's a very broad concept which is not only linked with the physical health or functioning of a person but also the psychological functioning of a person, his or her social relationships and relationship with environment also (WHO, 2005). According to psychology the well-being is linked with having a stable emotional and mental health, it is considered as an integral for good quality of life of an individual (López & Torres, 2001) in diverse contexts (Novoa-Gómez & Ballesteros, 2006).

From this perspective, psychological well-being is actually linked with the evaluation by a person in the light of his or her past, these evaluations also covers the way people reacted, behaved and made judgment. According to Diener, It's basically the view of a person by keeping in mind all dimensions of his or her life.

Many chronic diseases have their influence on every single sphere of one's life (Burish & Bradley, 1983). In acute disease, the life activities get effected temporally, whereas as in chronic illness there is a need to introduce temporary or permanent changes in one's life In addition, sufferers from the chronic illness must psychologically incorporate the role of a patient incase if they are to adapt to their disorders. As mentioned in the report of centers for disease control and prevention (2003) Dr. Venkat Narayan mentioned that "people are afraid when they first learn they have diabetes". After tension of diagnosis the patient started getting depressed and tense about the management of the disease. Furthermore, Dr. Narayan said the "you must deal with daily self-management of this disease". Then the very important and distressing thing is that diabetes can cause many problems which hinders the normal function of the individual like it start effecting the vision of the person and which in later stages turn into blindness, kidney diseases are very common, circulatory problems are also very common among diabetics and cognitive functioning also get declined. According to this report quality of life is worse in people with diabetes (CDC, 2007).

Soon after the diagnosis the patient is in a state of distress and have mostly imbalance in activities linked with all areas of their lives (physical, psychological and social). They figured out that their usual patterns of coping are not working. Their quality of life gets effected, therefore there is a need to get different treatment in order to get settle all the problems in the body or alter the functioning of some glands to have positive change in the body. The medical treatment has psychological impact, they produces the high level of stress and create uncertainty in patients. At that time there is a need to do a complete and proper psychological assessment of a patient (Ángel, as cited in Novoa, 2004; Luria, as cited in Grau & Pörtero, 1987).

Risk Factors

In the model proposed by Wallander and Varni (1989), the risk factors include three very important factors linked with the disease and its development. First, parameters which are linked with the disease or disability (for example, medical complications, cognitive impairments, visibility, diagnosis etc.). Second, dependency on others, related to daily living activities and third, stressors (psychosocial) (stressors like daily life events, disease or disability related problems). These all three major risk factors linked with the diseases or disabilities. Ultimately, this dependency was changed to independence by making minor changes in one's life (Wallander & Varni, 1998).

Risk factors included in the Transactional Stress and Coping Model includes two important but related factors. First, parameters linked with the illness i.e., type of disease and severity of the disease and second, parameters which are linked with the demography of an individual i.e., age, socio-economic status of an individual. Gold et al expanded the Transactional Stress and Coping Model in which they have further explained that parameters of illness are linked with the hospital visits of the person, whereas demographic factors include the information linked with siblings like gender, age, grade level and socio-economic status of siblings are included, the family factors are also included (e.g., extended family size).

Resistance Factors

Psychological factors sometimes indirectly influence behavior of the patients as according to some researchers the risk of cancer is indirectly linked with certain psychological factors which change the behaviors i.e., sleep, exercise, smoking, diet, poor adherence to medical regimens etc. (Cohen & Rodriquez, 1995; Spiegel & Kato, 1996). Risk factors are explained as psychosocial, environmental and biological risks, this will in turn increases the chances of adverse outcomes (Murray, 2003). These factors negatively affect the normal development and can increase the chances of adverse health outcomes. Risk factors can be eliminated and prevented. For prevention, multiple protective factors need to be explored. According to Haase (as cited in Huang, 2009), the protective or positive factors are explained as family, individual, contextual or social factors which promote the fighting back process and have positive outcomes. Protective factors can influence or change the impact of risk exposure and it can alter the health status of an individual. Furthermore, the affects of protective factors can be indirect in nature just like the risk factors (Huang, 2009). But in Murray's point of view the impact of the risk factors can be modified by the protective factors and in return it can change the health outcome status (Huang, 2009).

The risk factors i.e., age, duration of the disease, low social support, individual factors like defensive coping, and these factors directly affect the condition of the patients suffering from chronic illness (Haung, 2009). Social support is considered as a very important factor in altering the level of depression in cancer patients (Bailey et al., 2005). Low social support is considered as a risk factor for poor prognosis among heart patients (Compare et al., 2013). Individuals who are receiving more and more social support they show decrease in depression and other negative emotions or mood disturbances which are resulted because of illness (e.g., Brown, Nicassio, & Wallston, 1989). Lack of social support may affect the course and onset of cancer. The absence of close family ties in childhood may predict some cancer (Felitti et al., 1998). It is also predicted that the absence of social support network has been tied to a worsening of illness (Weihs, Enright, & Simmns, 2008). Coping strategies may influence the prognosis (Sprah & Sostaric, 2004). Furthermore, it has been identified that social support and coping strategies are related in predicting emotional well-being of women with cancer (Kim et al., 2011).

As there are different factors which are risk factors and they negatively affect the course of treatment such that few positive factors which plays a positive role in the good treatment of a patient. Social support has positive effect on physical and psychological well-being of people suffering from chronic illness such as cancer (Helgeson & Cohen, 1996). Social support affects the well-being of the patients (Swindells et al., 1999). Chronically ill patients use different coping strategies which help them in better and speedy recovery and with the use of active coping strategies produce more favorable outcomes such as less pain as well as depression, and better quality of life (Holmes & Stevenson, 1990). It has been reported that social support plays a moderating role in relationship between depressive symptoms and quality of life of cancer patients (Huang & Hsu, 2013).

Chronic illnesses contributed in the high mortality and disability rate. In the country like Pakistan about 42 percent of the deaths are because of chronic diseases. The burdens of chronic illnesses like cancer in which person not only have physiological constraints with him but also the deterioration of quality of life and work performance or sometimes discontinuation of the job (Short, Vasey, & Bellue, 2008).

Summing up the discussion, the chronically ill patients not only have physiological issues but also suffer from psychological ones and there is a need to address them. There are certain risk and protective factors which impact the psychological well-being and quality of life so there is a need to study these factors for the betterment of these patients.

Rationale of Study

The current study intended to address a vital issue of present time that health is not merely the absence of disease, it is in fact beyond it. Large number of chronically ill patients experiences many obstacles in dealing with their painful condition and unable to get the psychological support and information. Heath care programs are developed by the government to deal with all the issues related with the chronic illnesses (Wagner et al., 2014).

As literature has identified that patients who are suffering from the chronic diseases also suffer from the psychological issues like anxiety (Alter et al., 1999; Abraham, Degli-Esposti & Marino, 1999; Pariante, Orru, Baita, Farsi & Carpiniello, 1999), depression, hostility or aggression (Kraus et al., 2004; Ilic & Apostolovic, 2002), mood related problems and many of them suffer from other psychological problems (Turner & Brain, 2000). There is a need to provide them proper guidance and knowledge regarding their illness and outcomes of their illness. There is also a need to treat their psychological problems along with the physiological ones. As it is very much clear from the treatment plans that they only consider the physiological aspects of the treatment and they underestimate the impact of psychological issues on health, whereas the health gets deteriorated just because of these psychological issues.

It is important to explore the psychological issues of the chronically ill patients for their better treatment outcomes so it is very important for the healthcare professionals to identify those affected, ensure they receive appropriate care and provide ongoing support (Britneff & Winkley, 2013).

Psychological condition of the patients with chronic illness get effected and have worse the condition of the patients (Castera, Constant, Bernard, Ledinghen, & Couzigor, 2006; Hosoda et al., 1997; Kraus et al., 2004) but there is no single study which cater all the psychological problems and sometime one psychological issue can become the reason for another psychological disorder; so there is a need to study maximum psychological issues in one single study so that the proper consultancy will be provided timely and effectively. As discussed earlier, studies indicate that there is a direct association of declining physical status with mental-health. Studies indicated that the psychological adjustment or adaptation is very effective among chronically ill patients irrespective of their diagnosis (Cassileth et al., 1984).

As evident from the literature, few studies have focused on various psychological issue faced by chronically ill patients but these studies take these variables separately. There is a need to study multiple psychological issues simultaneously and also a need to evaluate the relationship between these issues. Furthermore, with reference to Pakistani patients, no significant researches have been conducted in this area. The present research aimed to fill in these gaps (study of psychological issues) in literature. Secondly in literature highlighted the psychological issues but psychological indicators are not explored there is a need to explore those psychological indicators.

It has also been observed that there are certain factors that may affect the relationship of psychological issues related to chronic illness. There are some risk factors such as age, duration of illness or disease, low social support, individual factors like defensive coping they may increase the likelihood of negative buffering effects of psychological issues on individual's mental and psychological functioning (Haung, 2009), whereas, some protective factors (i.e., social support and coping strategies) may intervene to save the individuals from these negative influences (i.e., depression, hopelessness, mood problems, sometime they commit suicide etc.) (Turner & Brian, 2000). Social support is figured out as a significant factor in lessening depression in cancer patients (Bailey et al., 2005). People who have received much social support have shown lower degrees of depression and other negative moods caused by physical illness (e.g. Brown, Nicassio & Wallston, 1989).

Coping strategies may influence the prognosis (Sprah & Sostaric, 2004). Furthermore, it has identified that social support and coping strategies are related in predicting emotional well-being of women with cancer (Kim et al., 2011). There are few important optimistic or positive factors which help in the good treatment of a patient. Social support has positive effect on physical and psychological well-being of people suffering from chronic illness such as cancer (Helgeson & Cohen, 1996). Social support affects the well-being of the patients (Swindells et al., 1999). Chronically ill patients use different coping strategies which help them in better and speedy recovery and with the use of active coping strategies patients can have a positive outcome like low level of depression and a good quality of life (Holmes & Stevenson, 1990).

Considering role of demographic variables (i.e., gender, education, marital status, age, family system and disease duration), literature suggests significant differences due to cultural effects. The socialization practices in Pakistan may assert gender-wise different roles in perception of stressful situations and coping strategies to deal with them. Other than gender, family system may also provide different scenario in our culture as compare to western societies. Those who are from the joint family system they share a strong and close bonding with one another. Whenever the support is needed it is always available and that is a very prominent feature of collectivistic culture. They expect a lot from one another that's why in case of any emergency or illness they come more and closer with one another (Cheema, Kaira & Bhugra, 2010). Another important factor is knowledge of patients about disease and course of treatment and it was identified through focus group discussions conducted for present study. It seems a cultural trend that patients are not disseminated detail information about their disease and prognosis. So role of demographic and contextual factors may depict unique patterns in Pakistani society. The focus is given upon to explore role of certain such variables in present study. Above all, present study has focused both risk and protective factors; which aggravate the symptoms and problems of chronically ill patients and those factors which increase the quality of life and wellbeing of a person.

In developing countries, the social and psychological conditions are worst (WHO, 2012). As in Pakistan there are few researches on the chronically ill patients and very few on psychological conditions of the patieqnts so present study is an effort to investigate the psychological issues which are experienced by chronically ill patients i.e., cardiovascular disease and diabetic patients. Cancer is a chronic disease and is the second leading cause of death in U.S (Bal & Foerster, 1991). The implications of conducting present study are twofold: it will not only help the specialists to treat their patients properly and in a more effective manner; But It will also help the professionals in considering preventive factors as interventions to facilitate the chronically ill patients.

METHOD

Present study broadly intended to explore the most commonly reported psychological issues among chronically ill patients and to explore risk and protective factors with regard to their impact on well-being and quality of life of patients.

Objectives of the Study

Present study was comprised of following objectives.

1. To find out the psychological issues of chronically ill patients (including Cardiac, cancer, and diabetes patients).

2. To find out impact of psychological issues on quality of life and well-being of patients.

3. To find out the risk factors that may increase the likelihood of negative effects of psychological issues on chronically ill patients.

4. To find out the protective factors that may contribute in relationship of psychological issues and their impact on wellbeing and quality of life of patients.

5. To investigate the effects of demographic, social and familial variables (i.e., education, gender, family history, family system, marital status, disease status and stage).

Conceptual and Operational Definitions

Chronically ill patients. Chronically ill patients are operationalized as those individuals who are suffering from chronic diseases i.e., cardiac, cancer and diabetes, were hospitalized and had no comorbidity of any other disease. Chronic diseases are mostly characterized as diseases of long duration and are slow in progression.

Psychological well-being. It is operationally defined as the state in which person strive for the perfection in his or her life and reaching to its full potential. In the current study it was assessed with the help of Psychological Well-being Scale, originally developed by Ryff and Keyes (1995) and translated in Urdu by Ansari in 2010. High score on this instrument highlighted that the high level of one's well-being (psychological) and low indicated low level.

Dimentions of psychological wellbeing It has six dimensions, these are Self-acceptance which refers to the positive evaluation of oneself and one's past, Purpose in life related to the belief that life is meaningful and purposeful, Personal growth is the sense of continued growth and development as a person, positive relations with others is linked with the ability to have a significant relationship with others, environmental mastery basically highlights that whether the person is having the ability to manage surrounding world, autonomy is linked with the freedom or freewill.

Quality of life. Quality of life is operationally defined as person's perception of his or her life in context of culture, in which they are living in relation to his or her life goals, standards and expectations. In present study it was measured through WHO Quality of life Questionnaire Khalid and Kausar (2006). High score indicates the high quality of life and low scores indicates low level of quality of life.

Dimentions of quality of life It has four dimensions, which includes physical functioning (individual is physically fully functioning and is not having any pain, discomfort issue and have optimal level of functioning), psychological functioning (deals with the positive feelings, thinking, learning, memory and concentration etc.), social relationships (deals with the functioning of individual in relation to their personal relationships, social support and sexual relationships), environment (functioning of the individual in home environment, financial resources, health and social care, physical environment etc.) and perception of quality of life (deals with the overall perception of individual about his or her quality of life).

Research Design

Current study was comprised of two parts.

Part – I. Part- I of the study divided into three phases. The Phase – I was dealing with the finalization of study variables (to identify psychological issues, their risk and protective factors) through focus groups and in-depth interviews, the Phase – II consisted of the Instrument development and the Phase – III dealt with determining the relibilities of study measures.

Part II. Part II was main study. Main objective was to test the study hypotheses. The specific objectives were to identify the most commonly reported psychological issues among chronically ill patients. It also explored the risk factors and protective factors linked with the chronic diseases. Then the relationship between the risk factors and protective factors were assessed with quality of life and well-being of the chronically ill patients. Furthermore, in the present study relationship between these variables with demographic variables was also explored.

Chapter III

PART-I

Part- I of the study encompassed three phases. Phase I dealt with the identification of psychological issues, their risk and protective factors through focus groups and in-depth interviews, Phase –II comprised of the Instrument development and Phase – III dealt with establishment of the relibilities of the instruments.

Phase – I: Identification of Psychological Issues, Risk & Protective Factors

Phase – I of Part-I of the study deals with the identification of psychological issues, risk and protective factors among chronically ill patients.

The Phase – I comprised of following stages.

Stage I. Focus group discussions were conducted by using multi-informant approach. In which the focus group discussions were conducted with the patients, doctors, nurses and caregivers of patients.

In order to explore most commonly reported psychological issues, the risk and protective factors, overall 30 focus groups were carried out. Each group was comprised of 6-9 members each.

Objectives. Focus Group Discussions (FGDs) were conducted to meet the following objectives.

1. To investigate the most commonly reported psychological issues among chronically ill patients.

2. To identify the factors that may play the role as risk factors for psychological issues.

3. To identify those factors that may play role as protective factors for psychological issues.

Focus group discussion (FGD). The FGDs were conducted by using multi-informant approach in which FGDs were conducted with patients, caregivers, doctors, nurses and para-medical staff, to explore the most commonly reported psychological issues among chronically ill patients, risk and protective factors linked with them. FDG's were conducted to get the first hand information about the most commonly reported psychological issues among chronically ill patients. 6 focus group discussions were conducted with patients, 6 with caregivers of the patients, 6 with doctors, 6 with nurses and paramedical staff.

Participants. For the focus group discussions patients, nurses, doctors, paramedical staff and caregivers were approached. 43 patients (16 cancer patients, 13 diabetic patients and 14 cardiac patients were taken from the Oncology, general medicine and Cardiology wards, Pakistan Institute of Medical Sciences, Islamabad (PIMS), 48 caregivers (17 caregivers of diabetic and cancer patients, 12 caregivers of cardiac patients), 35 nurses and 16 paramedical staff members and 33 doctors (21 females and 12 males) were approached. With the willingness of the participants they were included in the FGDs.

Inclusion criteria. Those patients who were suffering from other physiological diseases or psychological disorders were excluded from the study (those were included who were only suffering from one chronic disease at a time). Caregivers, doctors, nurses and para medical staff, who have direct interaction with the patients were included in study. Patients, caregivers, doctors, nurses and para medical staff was taken from PIMS hospital. Hospital authorities permitted then after this patient were approached. Then with the consent of the participants the data was collected.

Exclusion criteria. Patients suffering from two or more diseases at a time were excluded. Those who are in critical condition and cannot communicate were also excluded. Caregivers, doctors, nurses and para-medical staff who were not directly interacting with the patients were also excluded.

Focus group guide. On the basis of the extensive literature review (Crane, 1981; Dahlem, & Deffenbacher, 2001), Self-determination (Deci & Ryan, 2002), Diathesis – stress model (Ingram & Luxton, 2005) and the Disability-Stress-Coping

Model (Wallander & Varni, 1998) focus group guides (for patients, caregivers, doctors, nurses and paramedical staff) were prepared (see Annexure-A).

The categories explored through FGDs were chronic illness, change in behavior, emotions, cognition and feelings of the patients, along with them the risk and protective factors associated with the chronic illness.

Procedure. The patients, caregivers, doctors, nurses and para-medical staff were approached with the permission of the hospital authorities. The consent was taken from the participants and with their willingness they have participated in the study. These focus groups were conducted in the side room of the wards. The well trained moderator was accompanying by the well trained note taker and observer in the focus group discussion. After describing confidentiality measures the session was started. It took almost one hour and forty-five minutes to complete each focus group. The focus group discussions sessions were conducted with introductions and then followed by asking generally how they are feeling then the respondents were asked to state their condition by keeping in mind the disease. Then they were asked about their chronic condition. Firstly, the topic to be addressed was introduced and then the respondents were asked to briefly discuss their various conditions and symptoms. Next the respondents discussed the psychological issues faced by the patients and what are the risk and protective factors which are playing significant role in it.

In the end of every session the moderator summarized the major points and in the end of every focus group discussion the respondents were asked to add any information they believed to be important and to comment on the accuracy of reflection. The best efforts were made to have as homogeneous group as possible. A series of FGDs were conducted till no new information was generated and saturation point had reached. The order of putting the question was rotated in every focus group, so that the order effect on the responses of the participants could be minimized. The same procedure was adopted for conducting FGDs with caregivers, doctors, nurses and paramedical staff.

Focus group discussions with patients. The first 6 FGDs were conducted in the PIMS, Islamabad with chronically ill patients. These patients were suffering from cancer (taken from Oncology department of PIMS), Diabetes (taken from the General medicine department of PIMS) and cardiac patients (taken from the cardiology department of PIMS). Patients belong to lower SES (socio-economic status) and were married.

Participants. In order to conduct FGDs 43 patients (16 cancer patients, 13 diabetic patients and 14 cardiac patients were taken from the Oncology, general medicine and Cardiology wards of department of PIMS were approached. With their willingness they have taken a part in the discussions. Six FGDs were conducted to explore the most commonly reported psychological issues, risk and protective factors related with the chronic illness.

Focus group discussion I. Focus group one comprised of 7 cancer patients (4 females and 3 males) they were approached in the ward of Oncology Department, PIMS. Age ranges from 25-63 years. Patients belong to lower SES (socio-economic status) and were married.

Focus group discussion II. Focus group two comprised of 9 cancer patients (5 females and 4 males). Age ranges from 25-60 years. They were approached in the ward of Oncology Department, PIMS.

Focus group discussion III. Focus group three comprised of 6 diabetic patients (4 females and 2 males). Age ranges from 25-60 years. They were taken from the general medicine department of PIMS.

Focus group discussion IV. Focus group four comprised of 7 diabetic patients (5females and 2 males). Age ranges from 25-60 years. They were taken from the general medicine department of PIMS.

Focus group discussion V. Focus group five comprised of 6 cardiac patients (3females and 3 males). Age ranges from 25-60 years. They were taken from the ward of Cardiology department of PIMS.

Focus group discussion VI. Focus group six comprised of 8 cardiac patients (5females and 3 males). Age ranges from 25-60 years. They were taken from the ward of Cardiology department of PIMS.

Focus Group Discussion with Caregivers. The 6 focus group discussions were performed with the caregivers (including male and female members of the family) of the patients. The first 6 FGDs were conducted in the PIMS, Islamabad with caregivers of chronically ill (diabetic, cancer and cardiac) patients. These patients belong to lower socio economic status and were all married. These caregivers spend most of their time with the patients. Most of these caregivers were their children, siblings or parents.

*Participants.*48 caregivers (17 caregivers of diabetic and cancer patients, 12 caregivers of cardiac patients) were approached for the focus group discussions. With the willingness of the participants, they have participated. Six focus groups were performed in order to findout the most commonly reported psychological issues, risk and protective factors related with the chronic illness.

Focus group discussion I. Focus group one comprised of 8 caregivers of Cancer patient's (5 females and 3 males) they were approached in the ward of Oncology Department, PIMS, Islamabad. Age ranges from 20-40 years. They were from lower socio economic status. They were taking care of their relative and were mostly the children, sibling or parent of the patient.

Focus group discussion II. Focus group two comprised of 9 caregivers of Cancer patient's (5 females and 4 males) in second focus group. Age ranges from 20-40 years. They were approached in the ward of Oncology Department, PIMS. They were taking care of their relative and were mostly the children, sibling or parent of the patient.

Focus group discussion III. Focus group three comprised of 9 caregivers of diabetic patients (4 females and 5 males). Age ranges from 25-55 years. They were taken from the general medicine department of PIMS. They were taking care of their relative and were mostly the children, sibling or parent of the patient.

*Focus group discussion IV .*Focus group four comprised of 8 caregivers (4 females and 4 males) of diabetic patients. Age ranges from 25-55 years. They were taken from the general medicine department of PIMS. They were taking care of their relative and were mostly the children, sibling or parent of the patient.

Focus group discussion V. Focus group five comprised of 6 care givers of cardiac patients (3females and 3 males). Age ranges from 25-60 years. They were taken from the ward of Cardiology department of PIMS. They were taking care of their relative and were mostly the children, sibling or parent of the patient.

Focus group discussion VI. Focus group six comprised of 8 care givers of cardiac patients (5females and 3 males). Age ranges from 25-60 years. They were taken from the ward of Cardiology department of PIMS. They were taking care of their relative and were mostly the children, sibling or parent of the patient.

Focus group discussions with doctors. 6 focus groups were conducted with doctors, those who were treating the patients and dealing with them on daily basis. These were all experienced doctors and treating chronically ill patients from last eight to ten years. For the exploration of the psychological issues, risk and protective factors it was important to conduct focus group discussions with the doctors as they closely observe the patients.

*Participants.*33 doctors (21 females and 12 males) were approached for the focus group discussions. With the willingness of the participants, they were included in FGDs. Six FGDs were carried out in order to investigate the most commonly reported psychological issues, risk and protective factors related with the chronic illness.

Focus group discussion I. Focus group one comprised of 4 doctors (3 females and 1 male) they were approached in the ward of Oncology Department, PIMS, Islamabad. Age ranges from 25-40 years. They were specialized in treating cancer patients. Most of them were working with the patients from last 5-6 years.

Focus group discussion II. Focus group two comprised of 5 doctors (3 females and 2 males). Age ranges from 30-40 years. They were approached in the ward of Oncology Department, PIMS. They were specialized in treating cancer patients. Most of them were working with the patients from last 5-6 years.

Focus group discussion III. Focus group three comprised of 5 doctors (4 females and 1 male). Age ranges from 30-40 years. They were taken from the general medicine department of PIMS. They were specialized in treating diabetic patients. These doctors were working with these patients from last 5 years.

Focus group discussion IV. Focus group four comprised of 6 doctors (3 females and 3 males). Age ranges from 30-40 years. They were taken from the general medicine department of PIMS. They were specialized in treating diabetic patients. These doctors were working with these patients from last 5 -6 years.

Focus group discussion V. Focus group five comprised of 6 doctors (4females and 2 males). Age ranges from 25-46 years. They were taken from the ward of Cardiology department of PIMS. They were specialized in treating cancer patients. These doctors were working with these patients from last 5 years.

Focus group discussion VI. Focus group six comprised of 7 doctors (4 females and 3 males) in second focus group. Age ranges from 27-45 years. They were taken from the ward of Cardiology department of PIMS. They were specialized in treating cancer patients. These doctors were working with these patients from approximately last 5.

Focus group discussions with nurses and paramedical staff. 6 FGDs were conducted with nurses and paramedical staff, those who were dealing with patients from last at least 6 months. These were all those who were working with chronically ill patients from last so many years. For the exploration of the psychological issues, risk and protective factors it was important to conduct focus group discussions with the nurses and paramedical staff as they closely observe the patients.

*Participants.*35 nurses and 16 paramedical staff members were approached for the FGDs. With the willingness of the participants, they were included in the FGD. They were requested to share opinions. Six focus groups were performed in order to findout the most commonly reported psychological issues, risk and protective factors related with the chronic illness.

Focus group discussion I. Focus group one comprised of 5 female nurses and 4 paramedical staff members they were approached in the ward of Oncology Department, PIMS, Islamabad. Age ranges from 25-40 years. They were specialized in treating cancer patients.

Focus group discussion II. Focus group two comprised of 6 female nurses and 3 paramedical staff members. Age ranges from 25-40 years. They were approached in the ward of Oncology Department, PIMS. They were specialized in treating cancer patients.

Focus group discussion III. Focus group three comprised of 6 nurses and 6 paramedical staff members. Age ranges from 27-45 years. They were taken from the general medicine department of PIMS. They were specialized in treating cancer patients.

Focus group discussion IV. Focus group four comprised of 5 nurses and 5 paramedical staff members. Age ranges from 30-40 years. They were taken from the general medicine department of PIMS. They were specialized in treating cancer patients.

Focus group discussion V. Focus group five comprised of 6 nurses and 6 paramedical staff members (4females and 2 males). Age ranges from 25-38 years. They were taken from the ward of Cardiology department of PIMS. They were specialized in treating cancer patients.

Focus group discussion VI. Focus group six comprised of 7 nurses and 7 paramedical staff members (4 females and 3 males) in second focus group. Age ranges from 27-45 years. They were taken from the ward of Cardiology department of PIMS. They were specialized in treating cancer patients.

Stage 2: Content analysis of focus group data of patients, caregivers, doctors, nurses and paramedical staff. The data was organized, coded separately and then themes were generated through content analysis approach (Berelson, 1952). The process includes the open coding, in which the information was read again and again to gain insight into the data. While reading the notes, the headings were written, many headings were created. These all headings were clearly describing all the aspects of the data. In the next step all these headings were taken to the code sheet. Then the categories were generated at that stage. After the coding of the data the list of the categories were grouped under the high order headings. The main objective behind this grouping was actually to reduce the number of categories by organizing the categories and grouping the categories into similar and dissimilar ones. This all was done not just to group together the similar and non-similar information, basically it was done to describe the phenomenon, to having insight into it and to generate knowledge out of it. Themes were generated with the help of content analysis method. The major themes were generated by the committee of judges. The themes were as follow.

Table 1

Themes and Indicators or Statements of Patients, Doctors, Caregivers, Nurses and paramedical staff for Psychological Issues, Risk and Protective Factors

Themes	Statements or indicators
Psychological Issues	بہت نا امیدی ہے۔
	اپنے آپ سے تنگ ہوں۔
	دل کرتا ہے کہ دنیا چھوڑ دوں۔
	کسی چیز میں دل نہیں لگتا۔
	کھانے پینے کو دل نہیں کرتا۔
	نیند بھی جیسے ختم ہی ہو گئی ہے۔ ساری رات پڑی رہتی ہوں پر نیند نہیں آتی۔
	بہت اُداسی ہے۔
	اکیلے رہنے کا دل کرتا ہے۔
	کسی سے بات کرنے کا بھی دل نہیں کرتا۔
	لگتا ہے جیسے زندگی ختم ہوگئی ہے۔
	سب کچھ جیسے ختم ہوگیا ہوں۔
	کبھی کبھی سمجھ نہیں آتی کے کیا ہوگا۔
	اس طرح دوسروں کے بھروسے رہنے سے اچھا ہے کہ مر ہی جاؤ۔
Psychological issues	بہت غصہ آتا ہے۔

کبھی کبھی دل کرتا ہے کہ چیزیں اٹھا اٹھا کے پٹخوں۔

پہلے کبھی اتنا غصہ نہیں آتا تھا جتنا اب آتا ہے۔

اب ہر چھوٹی چھوٹی بات پر غصہ آتا ہے۔

بے وجہ غصہ کرنے لگی ہوں۔

کبھی کبھی کنٹرول ہوتا ہے اور کبھی کبھی نہیں۔

اب کنٹرول مشکل لگتا ہے۔

Risk and Protective Factors

جس دن اپنے گھر والوں سے ملوں تو طبیعت بہتر ہوتی ہے۔

اپنی فیملی کے لیے ٹھیک ہونا چاہتی ہوں۔

بچوں کی وجہ سے ٹھیک ہونا چاہتی ہوں۔

بیٹوں کو دیکھ کے زندگی کی طرف آ جاتی ہوں۔

جب اپنے ساتھ نہیں دیتے تو دل کرتا ہے کہ دنیا چھوڑ دوں۔

مشکل حالات میں کبھی کبھی اپنے ساتھ دیتے ہیں تو اچھا محسوس ہوتا ہے۔

جب انسان بیمار ہوتا ہے تو کوئی ہی اسے پوچھتا ہے۔ خوش نصیب ہے وہ جسے کوئی پوچھنے آئے۔

کچھ خاندان کے لوگ بہت ہمت افزائی کرتے ہیں۔

میرے بچے مجھے ہر حال میں اہمیت دیتے ہیں۔

ایسا لگتا ہے جیسے بیماری کے بعد لوگ مجھے چھوڑ گئے ہیں۔

Risk and Protective Factors

اللہ پر یقین ہے کہ میں ٹھیک ہوں جاوں گی۔

بس اللہ پر بھروسہ ہے۔

جب بھی دل اداس ہوتا ہے تو اللہ کو یاد کروں تو بہتر محسوس کرتا ہوں۔

خدا کو یاد کر کے سکون ملتا ہے۔

کبھی کبھی خدا سے بھی یقین اٹھ جاتا ہے۔

سمجھ میں نہیں آتا کہ کیا ہوگا۔

کبھی کبھی سب کچھ چھوڑ دینے کا دل کرتا ہے۔

جب زیادہ پریشان ہوتا ہوں تو اپنے آپ کو کسی اور کام میں لگا لیتا ہوں۔

Table 1 indicates that the statements for each theme. It is basically providing the participants conceptual understanding about psychological issues, risk and protective factors.

Table 2

Themes and Sub Themes Related to Psychological Issues, Risk and Protective Factors

Themes	Subthemes
Sleep issues	Sleeplessness
Appetite issues	Loss of appetite
Loss of interest	Loss of interest in life activities
	Irritability
Sadness	Feel like crying
	Restlessness
	All the time sadness
Anger on small issues	Reacting quickly and violently to small problems
	Getting violent on pity matters
	Feel like anger is not under control
Hitting or beating others	Feel like hitting other
	Shout loudly
	Hit others
	Feeling angry
	Finding it difficult to calm the feeling of anger
Religious coping strategies	Praying
	Faith in Allah Almighty
	Small ray of hope
Distractive strategies	Started meeting people and going to social gatherings

	Distracting mind with different activities
	Indulging in some activity
	Not thinking about the problem
Avoidance coping strategies	tried forgetting for the event which has happened
	avoiding others
practical coping strategies	Going to doctors
	Meeting professionals to seek help related to disease
	wanted professional help for the solution of problem
	Seeking knowledge linked with the disease
	Asking for help linked with disease
	Reading books or brouchers linked with the disease
Help or support of others	Support of the caregivers
	Support of family
	Family's interest in health
	Family's response
Lack of Social support	Negative attitude of family
	Family's negligence

Themes were generated through the content analysis, which include sadness, crying spells, sleeping difficulty, hopelessness, loss of interest in life, appetite problems and loss of interest in everything, physical and verbal aggression as major indicators of psychological issues. So most of the chronically ill patients suffer from the psychological problems and the signs and symptoms were very clear. High and low social support and different coping strategies were highlighted as a risk and protective factors. Furthermore, it was also highlighted that the low level of social support, distractive and avoidance coping strategies are risk factors. And high levels of social support, practical and religious focused coping strategies were protective factors.

After the data analysis by the researcher the committee approach was conducted. This committee of experts revisited the statements and themes. This committee comprised of 2 health psychologists, 2 M. Phil and 2 Ph. D (psychology) scholars. They have extensive knowledge about the psychological issues about chronically ill patients and qualitative research. They first independently gone through the statements and themes and then it was checked that whether they all have consensus on the given themes or not. It was found that they have consensus on all the given themes. To explore the inter-rater reliability Krippendorff's alpha was explored as it is the standard reliability statistic (inter-rater reliability) for content analysis and similar data (Hayes & Krippendorff, 2007). Its .87 which is high reliability, it indicates that the six coders have consensus on the themes.

Discussion. The present phase of the resent study was carried out to findout the psychological issues, risk and protective factors among patients (chronically ill). In this phase of study, the FGDs were conducted to find out the psychological issues, risk and protective factors among chronically ill patients.

Worldwide, the main reason behind death and disability is chronic illnesses or diseases. In Pakistan, fourty two percent of all the deaths are caused because of chronic diseases or illness. The burden not only include the illnesses like cancer but the pateints also have to face the deterioration of the health but also the disability in working and adverse quality of life (Short, Vasey, & Bellue, 2008). In this part of study, the multi-informant approach was used to provide a broader and clear picture about psychological issues, risk and protective factors because it is assumed that patients sometimes exaggerate the problems and sometimes cannot properly report their problems so it is necessary to get the information from some other sources.

Literature highlighted that most of the researches done on exploration of psychological issues are either done only with patients (Anderston, Freedland, Clouse, & Lustman, 2001; Lewko & Misiak, 2015; Solowiejczyk, 2010) or the caregivers or the doctors (Mitnick, Leffler, & Hood, 2009), there is a less research on having all these perspectives (patients, caregivers, doctors, nurses and paramedical staff) under one umbrella of research. There is a need to have a research which explains the psychological issues of chronically ill patients, risk and protective factors by having the perspectives of all informants by using multi-informant approach, including patients themselves, doctors, caregivers, nurses and paramedical staff.

In order to have a complete and detailed picture of the psychological issues, risk and protective factors among chronically ill patients the FGDs were conducted. On the basis of the literature review (Crane, 1981; Dahlem & Deffenbacher, 2001), and different theoretical models i.e., Self-determination (Deci & Ryan, 2002), Diathesis – stress model (Ingram & Luxton, 2005) and the Disability-Stress-Coping Strategy (Wallander & Varni, 1998) focus group guides for caregivers, patients, nurses, paramedical staff and doctors were prepared. Probing questions were also generated under each question for getting a breath of responses. FGD guides covered different categories i.e., chronic illness, change in behavior, emotions, cognition and feelings of the patients associated with the chronic illness.

After FGD the data was analyzed with the content analysis method. The data was ordered, systematized, separately coded and after that the themes were generated through content analysis approach, which is widely used to have a detailed and in-depth analysis of qualitative data (Berelson, 1952). Through the analysis the most commonly reported psychological issues were highlighted. The themes were loss of interest in life, sleeping difficulty, appetite problems crying spells, sadness, hopelessness, and loss of interest in everything aggression (both, physical & verbal). Literature also indicates that these issues are common among chronically ill patients (Anderston, Freedland, Clouse, & Lustman, 2001; Lewko & Misiak, 2015; Solowiejczyk, 2010). Furthermore, the data revealed that the indicator of hopelessness is identified by patients, caregivers, doctors, nurses and paramedical staff. Crying spells and difficulty falling in sleep were identified by patients and caregivers. Loss of interest and irritability is identified by patients, caregivers, doctors, nurses and paramedical staff. Shouting and behaving aggressively was identified by patients themselves, caregivers, doctors, nurses and paramedical staff. Literature also highlighted that the chronic diseases increases the chances of severe psychological issues i.e., diabetes increases the risk of depression (Anderston, Freedland, Clouse, & Lustman, 2001) which are enlined with present study findings.

Results revealed that depressive feelings and feelings of anger are common among cardiac patients and literature also highlighted this fact (Ilic & Apostolovic, 2002; Solowiejczyk, 2010). Caregivers and doctors also mentioned that the patients have crying spills and develop hopelessness, in other words a depression. Depression is also reported by the caregivers of the chronically ill (cancer) patients (Taylor, 2006). Daughter of cancer patient reported that her father said that "let me alone. No more treatments" (cited in Taylor, 2006). According to doctors the patients are more in a hopeless condition and as one of the diabetic patient on doctor's suggestion she bursts out sadly and started crying and said to the doctor that "she has tried everything but nothing works" (Greenberg, 2007).

Anger sadness and guilt have been reported by these patients (Shapiro, 1996). In FGDs the results also clearly indicate feelings of hopelessness, crying spells and sad feelings. The most common psychiatric disorders in cancer patients are depression, anxiety disorders and adjustment disorders (Gregurek et al., 2010). These are the common issues with the chronically ill patients.

Literature indicates that chronically ill patients frequently use problem-focused coping strategies and sometimes use emotional focus coping strategies (Tuncay, Musabak, Gok, & Kutlu, 2008). In the present study results also revealed that some patients indulge in religious activities to deal with the psychological disorders they are suffering from, whereas some distract their mind by doing different other activities.

Stage 3: Interviews of patients, caregivers, doctors and nurses.

Objective. After the focus group discussion in order to have more detailed and complete information about the psychological issues, risk and protective factors, the in depth interviews were conducted by using the multi-informant approach.

Participants. 6 patients, 6 caregivers, 6 doctors and 6 nurses were interviewed.

Interview Guide. Literature (Anderston, Freedland, Clouse, & Lustman, 2001; Lewko & Misiak, 2015; Shapiro, 1996; Solowiejczyk, 2010) was explored and on the bases of focus group discussions, Self-determination (Deci & Ryan, 2002), Diathesis – stress model (Ingram & Luxton, 2005) and the Disability-Stress-Coping Strategy (Wallander & Varni, 1998) interview guidelines were prepared to interview patients, caregivers, doctors and nurses to identify the most commonly reported psychological issues, risk and protective factors (see Annexure-B).

Sample 1. Were conducted with 6 patients 2 were cancer patients, 2 diabetics and 2 cardiac patients. Age ranges from 25 years to 40 years.

Sample 2. For this purpose, 6 caregivers of patients (2 caregivers of cancer patients, 2 caregivers of diabetic and 2 caregivers of cardiac patients) were approached. Age ranges from 25 years to 40 years.

Sample 3. For this purpose, 6 doctors (2 from oncology department, 2 from general medicine and 2 from the cardiology department). These were those doctors who were directly dealing with the patients and observing them from last 5 -6 years were approached and interviewed. Age ranges from 25 years to 40 years.

Sample 4. 6 nurses (2 from oncology department, 2 from general medicine and 2 from the cardiology department). These nurses were directly dealing with the patients. Age ranges from 30 years to 40 years.

Procedure. With the permission of the authorities the patients, caregivers, nurses and doctors were approached. Two patients were taken from the Oncology department, two were taken from the General Medicine and two from the Cardiology department. Those who were willing to participate were interviewed. Then the caregivers were interviewed. 6 caregivers of patients (2 caregivers of cancer patients, 2 caregivers of diabetic and 2 caregivers of cardiac patients) were approached. Then doctors were requested. Those who were free and gave the appointment were interviewed. 6 doctors (2 from oncology department, 2 from general medicine and 2 from the cardiology department) were interviewed. Then nurses were approached and 6 nurses (2 from oncology department, 2 from general medicine and 2 from the cardiology department) were interviewed. Those nurses, who were directly dealing with chronically ill patients.

Stage 4. Content analysis of interview data. Content analysis approach was used to analyze the interview data. The data was organized, coded separately and then themes were generated through content analysis approach (Berelson, 1952). The themes were generated from interview data, with the help of content analysis method. So firstly the data was transcribed and then organized. Then the open coding was done by reading the material again and again. While reading the text the notes, the headings were written on the same page. The headings were actually summarizing the information and also provided the sort of theme for specific information. In the next step the headings were written on for the coding purpose and then the data was coded. After the coding of the data the list of the categories were grouped under the high order headings. So the numbers of the categories were generated. Now the data was grouped in form categories. These categories were basically describing the phenomenon. The major themes were generated by the committee of judges. On the basis of the interviews themes were emerged by content analysis approach.

Results. The information gathered through the interviews was analyzed in detailed manner and then the themes were generated. Through the analysis the most commonly reported psychological issues were highlighted and risk and protective factors among chronically ill patients

Table 3

Themes and Indicators or Statements of Patients, Doctors, Caregivers, Nurses and paramedical staff for Psychological Issues, Risk and Protective Factors

Themes	*Statements or indicators*
Psychological issues	مریض بہت خاموش رہتے ہیں۔
	جینا ہی نہیں چاہتے۔
	کبھی کبھی بہت غصہ کرتے ہیں۔
	ان کا موڈ کافی ڈاون ہوتا ہے۔
	بہت ڈپرس رہتے ہیں۔
	کوئی کام کرنے کا دل نہیں کرتا۔

غصہ برداشت نہیں ہوتا۔

غصہ کرتے ہیں۔

بلاوجہ غصہ کرتے ہیں۔

Risk and protective factors   جس دن رشتے دار آتے ہیں اُس دن ٹھیک اور خوش نظر آتے ہیں۔

ان کو پیار دیا جائے تو ٹھیک اور خوش نظر آتے ہیں۔

کچھ کے رشتے دار بھی اب اس بیماری سے تھک چکے ہیں جس کی وجہ سے وہ اب ان پر توجہ

نہیں دیتے ہیں۔ اور کچھ میں یہ کافی یقین ہے کہ ان کے مریض نے نہیں بچنا اس لیے بھی

وہ ہمت ہار چکے ہیں۔

اپنے بچوں کی خاطر ٹھیک ہونا چاہتی ہوں۔

بیماری میں سب چھوڑ جاتے ہیں۔

خاندان والے بوجھ سمجھتے ہیں۔

کچھ مریض بہت خاموش رہتے ہیں۔

کچھ مریض دین کے بہت نزدیک ہوجاتے ہیں۔

کچھ یہ سوچتے ہیں کہ ٹھیک تو ہونا نہیں تو اس لیے علاج کا فائدہ۔

کچھ مریض اپنے آپ کو کسی اور کام/سرگرمیوںمیں مصروف کر لیتے ہیں۔

    Table 3 comprised of patient's interview statements. The data was organized, coded separately and then themes were generated through content analysis approach (Berelson, 1952). The focus group discussion data indicated these themes were hopelessness, crying spells, sleeping difficulty, loss of interest in life, sadness, appetite problems and loss of interest in everything, physical and verbal aggression as major indicators of psychological issues. Whereas the major indicators of the risk and protective factors are social support and coping strategies (active-practical coping, active-distractive coping, avoidance-focused coping and religious-focused coping).

After the data analysis by the researcher the committee approach was conducted. This committee of experts revisited the statements and themes. This committee comprised of 2 health psychologists and 2 Ph. D (psychology) scholars. They have extensive knowledge about the psychological issues about chronically ill patients and qualitative research. They first independently gone through the statements and themes and then it was checked that whether they all have consensus on the given themes or not. It was found that they have consensus on all the given themes. To explore the inter-rater reliability Krippendorff's alpha was explored as it is the standard reliability statistic (inter-rater reliability) for content analysis and similar data (Hayes & Krippendorff, 2007). It's .83 which is high reliability, which indicates that the four coders have consensus on the themes.

Stage 5. Committee approach for the finalization of study variables.

Objective. For the identification of psychological issues, risk and protective factors the committee approach was conducted

Results. The data generated through FGDs and in-depth interviews was analyzed through content analysis approach. The committee approach was conducted after the completion of content analysis. The data and themes extracted through the content analysis of FGDs and interview data was reviewed by the panel of experts. Expert's panel comprised of the two health psychologists and 3 practicing psychologists. They have critically viewed every single theme. Then they have mentioned the major themes and provided the researcher with the themes and subthemes. The experts have repeatedly reviewed the statements and then they have explained the clear categories which were indicated by the statements. These themes were depression and anger which were highlighted as a most commonly occurring psychological issue, whereas the coping strategies and social support are the factors which are considered as a risk and protective factor. After the committee approach the statements and themes generated were discussed with different experts and they have confirmed the themes, which were deduced from the data.

Table 4

Themes and Sub Themes for Psychological Issues, risk and protective factors among Chronically Ill Patients

Themes	Subthemes
	Sleeplessness
	Loss of appetite
Depression	Loss of interest in life activities
	Irritability
	Feel like crying
	Restlessness
	All the time sadness
Anger	Reacting quickly and violently to small problems
	Getting violent on pity matters
	Feel like anger is not under control
	Feel like hitting other
	Shout loudly
	Hit others
	Feeling angry
	Finding it difficult to calm the feeling of anger
Religious coping strategies	Praying
	Faith in Allah Almighty
	Small ray of hope
Active-distractive coping strategies	Started meeting people and going to social gatherings
	Distracting mind with different activities
	Indulging in some activity
	Not thinking about the problem
Avoidance-focused coping strategies	tried forgetting for the event which has happened
	avoiding others
Active-practical coping strategies	Going to doctors
	Meeting professionals to seek help related to disease
	wanted professional help for the solution of problem

	Seeking knowledge linked with the disease
	Asking for help linked with disease
	Reading books or broachers linked with the disease
Social support	Support of the caregivers
	Support of family
	Family's interest in health
	Family's response
Lack of Social support	Negative attitude of family
	Family's negligence

The themes generated through content analysis were hopelessness, crying spells, sleeping difficulty, loss of interest in life, sadness, appetite problems and loss of interest in everything, physical and verbal aggression as major indicators of psychological issues, whereas the major indicators of the risk and protective factors are social support and coping strategies. After the data analysis by the researcher the committee approach was conducted.

After detailed review of all the themes, two major disorders identified by the experts and these were depression and the anger. Social support and coping strategies were highlighted as a risk and protective factors. Furthermore, they have also highlighted low level of social support, active-distractive and avoidance-focused coping strategies as Risk factors. And high level of social support, active practical and religious focused coping strategies as Protective factors.

Discussion. The current study was carried out to explore the most commonly occurring psychological issues, risk and protective factors among patients (chronically ill). In this stage of the study, the interviews were conducted to get more detailed information about the psychological issues, risk and protective factors among patients (chronically ill), as the interviews are comparably rich source of data (Anderson & Arsenault, 2005). The interview guides were prepared with the help of the information collected through the focus group discussion, Diathesis – stress model (Ingram & Luxton, 2005), Self determination (Deci & Ryan, 2002) and the Disability-

Stress-Coping Strategy (Wallander & Varni, 1998). Separate interview guides were prepared for the patients, their caregivers, doctors and nurses. Almost same information was provided in the interviews. The doctors and nurses reported that the patients have lost all their hopes and are waiting for the death. Caregivers were also reporting that the patients have developed a wrong thinking that they are not going to recover. On the basis of in depth interviews various themes were emerged by content analysis approach. The themes were extracted through content analysis. For the content analysis the data was organized, coded and then the themes were generalized.

The results of the interviews also revealed that the incidence of anger among chronically ill patients. Anger, sadness and guilt have been mentioned and explained by these patients (Shapiro, 1996). The most common psychological issue in cancer patients are adjustment, anxiety and depression disorders (Gregurek et al., 2010). Numbers of chronically ill patients are increasing day by day and they find it extremely difficult to deal with issues related with them and unable to get the psychological support and information.

People use different coping strategies to deal with issues related to their illness. Literature indicates that chronically ill patients frequently use problem-focused coping strategies and sometimes use emotional focus coping strategies (Tuncay, Musabak, Gok, & Kutlu, 2008). Interview results revealed that some patients indulge in religious activities to deal with the psychological disorders they are suffering from, whereas some distract their mind by doing different other activities.

There are some risk factors such as age, duration of illness or disease, low social support, individual factors like defensive coping they may increase the likelihood of negative buffering effects of psychological issues on individual's mental and psychological functioning (Haung, 2009), whereas, some protective factors (i.e., social support and coping strategies) may intervene to save the individuals from these negative influences (i.e., depression, hopelessness, mood problems, sometime they commit suicide etc.) (Turner & Brian, 2000). Social support has been identified as an important factor alleviating depression in cancer patients (Bailey et al., 2005). Those who are getting high social support they experience low level of negative mood especially depression (Brown, Wallston, & Nicassio, 1989). There are some positive or protective or effective aspects which may help in the effective treatment of a patient. Social support has positive effect on physical and psychological well-being of people suffering from chronic illness such as cancer (Helgeson & Cohen, 1996). Social support affects the well-being of the patients (Swindells et al., 1999).

Coping strategies may influence the prognosis (Sprah & Sostaric, 2004). Chronically ill patients use different coping strategies which help them in better and speedy recovery and with the use of active coping strategies produce more favorable outcomes such as less pain as well as low level of depression, and better quality of life (Holmes & Stevenson, 1990). Furthermore, it has been identified that social support and coping strategies are related in predicting emotional well-being of women with cancer (Kim, Han, Shaw, Mctavish, & Gustafson, 2011). Literature also shows that psychological issues may impact negatively on the quality of life (Chen, Baungardner, & Rice, 2011; Vila et al., 2003) and psychological wellbeing of the patients (Dubey, 2012). Heath care programs are developed by the government to deal with all the issues related with the chronic illnesses (Wagner et al., 2014). It is important to explore the psychological issues of the chronically ill patients for their better treatment outcomes so it is very important for the healthcare professionals to identify those who got affected, ensure they receive appropriate care and provide ongoing support (Britneff & Winkley, 2013).

Conclusion. The content analysis of the information of the FGDs and indepth interviews revealed that the most commonly occurring psychological issues were depression and anger. The risk factor was the social support and it was also considered as a protective factor that if patient is getting it he or she will feel very good and have positive mood but if there is a low level of social support then it adversely affects their health. Along with the social support, the religious coping strategy and practical coping strategy was also considered as a protective factor as it helps them to cope with the problem, whereas the avoidance and distractive coping strategies are risk factors because it makes them to avoid everything.

Phase - II: Instrument Development

In Phase I variables for the present study were finalized. For psychological issues depression and anger are commonly reported by chronically ill patients, whereas the social support and coping strategies are figured out as a risk and protective factor. For the assessment of depression the Beck Depression Inventory (Khan, 1996) was used, Social Support Scale (Malik, 2002) for the assessment of social support, Coping Strategies Questionnaire (Kausar & Munir, 2004) for the assessment of coping strategies, WHO Quality of Life Questionnaire by Khalid and Kausar (2006) for the assessment of quality of life, Psychological wellbeing (Ansari, 2010) was used for the assessment of psychological well being and for the measurement of anger, the literature was investigated and previously developed questionnaires and inventory (Siegel, 1986; Speilberger, 1999) were reviewed. Most of the instruments were in English. No specific anger scale was there with which their (chronically patients) anger can be assessed. To develop the instrument which cover all domains and will be in Urdu, the new scale was developed. Many general scales were there which can be used either for healthy or unhealthy individuals; no specific scale was there for chronically ill patients. Secondly in order to have an indigenous scale for assessing anger of patients (chronically ill). The Phase – II deals with the development of the Anger Scale for Chronically ill Patients (ASCIP).

Stage-I: Development of Scale. It was dealing with the construction of ASCIP. In this stage the already developed scales were reviewed. Stage –I was comprised of following steps:

Step – I: Review of literature and previously developed scales. The wide research evidences about anger was reviewed before the development of (Crane, 1981; Dahlem & Deffenbacher, 2001), along with the literature review already developed scales (Siegel, 1986; Speilberger, 1999) were reviewed by expert committee which comprised of six PhD and six MPhil scholars. The indicators indentified in FGD's (conducted in Phase – I of present study) were also taken. The committee had detailed discussions on anger and its dimensions. With the help of these discussions they have gathered the content of the scale.

Step – II: Generation of Items pool and rating scale selection. This step was about having a committee approach. Objective of the committee approach was to construct or develop the item pool. This committee was consisted of six members, including three PhD and three MPhil scholars; they have wide knowledge of research and scale construction, also have its experience. The item-pool was generated with the help of literature review (Crane, 1981; Dahlem & Deffenbacher, 2001), critically analysis of already developed anger scales (Siegel, 1986; Speilberger, 1999) and a discussion with subject matter experts. Furthermore, the indicators highlighted in FGDs were also taken into consideration. On the basis of all that the dimensions for the scale were acquired and on their basis the items were written. 57 items were formulated and having a four-point response option of very much so, moderately so, somewhat and not at all.

Step III: Committee Approach for items selction. After extensive literature review, analysis of already developed scales, indicators highlighted in FGDs and discussions with SMEs the items were written. Item finalization was carried out in committee approach. This committee consisted of 3 MPhil scholars, 2 PhD scholars and 1 Associate professor (taken from NIP, QAU, Islamabad). Thus with the help of their expert opinion the items were critically analyzed so they become free from any flow. The items were checked for difficulty, double-barrel and mislead. All items were considered appropriate by the committee. The item pool of ASCIP was comprised of 57 items (see Annexure-C). In the committee approach the 25 items were finalized.

After finalization of the items, the scale was ready for tryout. The tryout was conducted by taking twenty participants and administering scale on them. Participants were requested to provide their feedback about the ASCIP. They all were appealed to mention, in case they got any perplexity or complexity in understanding any item or if there is any doubt or vagueness in anything. After the completion of questionnaire, the respondents were asked about the scale and they have mentioned that they have easily filled it up.

Stage – II: Exploration of factors for ASCIP.

Objective. The main objective of this stage was to explore factor analysis of the ASCIP.

Sample. The sample comprised of 300 chronically ill patients (cancer, diabetic and cardiac patients), taken from Oncology, cardiology and General Medicine Department of PIMS. Both female and male participants were taken. They were all diagnosed patients. Those having to illness at a time or having any psychological disorder were excluded.

Table 5

Descriptive Characteristics of the Sample (N=300)

Variables	f	$\%$	M	SD
Disease				
Diabetes	100	33.3		
Cancer	100	33.3		
Cardiac	100	33.3		
Duration of illness			13.64	11.92
Stage of disease				
Stage 4 (Cancer)	100	33.3		
Cardiac (first heart attack)	100	33.3		
Diabetes (High & Insulin dependent)	100	33.3		
Gender				
Male	91	30.3		
Female	209	69.7		
Age			31.95	13.81
Education				
Un educated	87	29.0		
Primary	34	11.3		

Middle	19	6.3
Matric	62	20.7
FA/F.Sc	40	13.3
BA/B.Sc	54	18.0
M.Sc	4	1.3
Marital Status		
Married	198	66.0
Unmarried	102	34.0
Family system		
Nuclear	175	58.3
Joint	125	41.7
Employment Status		
Employed	46	15.3
Unemployed	254	84.7
Monthly Income in Rupees		
Less than 10000	142	47.3
Between 10000 – 50000	142	47.3
Above 50000	16	5.3

Table 5 explains about the descriptive characteristics of the study sample. This part of study was consisted of 300 chronically ill patients (100 diabetics, 100 cardiac and 100 cancer patients). Male and female both patients were taken. 175 belong to nuclear family and 125 belong to joint families.

Procedure. Chronically ill patients were approached after taking the consent from the hospital authorities. The cardiac patients, cancer and diabetic patients were taken from Cardiology, Oncology and general medicine department of the PIMS hospital. With the willingness of the patients the data was collected. The purpose of the study was mentioned to them. Furthermore, they were also explained about their right to reject and withdraw at any point of time. Approximately in an hour they have completed the questionnaire. Along with the questionnaire the demographic information was also acquired, it included information about gender, occupation, age, marital status, stage of illness, duration of illness etc. As they were chronically ill so they were taking pauses while completing the questionnaire, there comfort was assured and maintained. All other ethical guidelines which were provided by the American Psychological Association were followed.

    Results. For the computation of the fators or dimensions of the scale, the items were analyzed on Exploratory Factor Analysis (EFA). EFA was computed in order to explore the factors of the scale. On Principal component and by using the varimax rotation the factors were extracted. As varimax rotation is most widely and commonly used for orthogonal rotataion, when the factors are not related with one another (Brown, 2009). By using Factor, the EFA was computed (Ferrando & Lorenzo-Seva, 2016). The Kaiser-Meyer-Olkin (KMO) test value is .71.

Table 6

Factor Loadings and EigenValues of Items of ASCIP (N = 300)

Items		F1	F2	F3	F4	F5
4	میرا کسی کو مارنے کادل کرتا ہے۔	.95				
3	میں غصے سے پاگل ہوں۔	.95				
7	میرا دل اُونچی آواز میں لعن طعن کرنے کو کرتا ہے۔	.95				
2	میرا غصے سے چلانے کو جی چاہتا ہے۔	.95				
6	میرا دل کسی کو ٹھوکر مارنے کوکرتا ہے۔	.94				
8	میرا کسی پر حملہ کرنے کو جی کرتا ہے۔	.93				
5	میں سخت ناراض محسوس کرتی/کرتا ہوں۔	.88				
25	میں اُس سے کئی زیادہ چڑچڑا ہوتا ہوں جتنا لوگ سمجھتے ہیں۔	.83				
9	میرا باآوازبلند چلانے کو جی کرتا ہے۔	.81				
1	میں چڑچڑا ہوں۔	.75			.50	

Item No.	Statement	F1	F2	F3	F4
13	جب میں غصے سے پاگل ہوتی ہوں تو گھٹیا باتیں کہتی ہوں۔	.61			.50
20	میں دوبارہ پُرسکون ہونے کی کوشش کرتا/کرتی ہوں۔		.93		
17	میں پُر سکون اور پُر آمن رہنے کی کوشش رہنے کی کوشش کرتا/کرتی ہوں۔		.90		
21	میں خود کو بے قابو ہونے سے روک سکتی/سکتاہوں۔		.88		
18	میں خود کو پُر سکون رکھتی ہوں۔		.86		
22	میں اپنے غصے کو جتنی جلدی ممکن ہوسکے کم کرتا/کرتی ہوں۔		.84		
19	میں اپنے غصے والے احساسات کو پُرسکون رکھنے کی کوشش کرتا/کرتی ہوں۔		.78		
11	میں بہت گرم دماغ آدمی ہوں۔		.77		
10	میں بہت جلد غصے میں آجاتی/آجاتا ہوں۔		.60		
15	میں دوسروں کے ساتھ صبر و تحمل سے پیش آتی ہوں/آتا ہوں۔			.89	
12	میں یکدم آپے سے باہر ہوجاتا ہوں/ہوجاتی ہوں۔			.89	
23	جتنا میں مانتی ہوں میں اُس سے کئی زیادہ غصہ کرتی ہوں۔			.89	
24	میں اپنے غصے کے احساسات کو قابو میں کرتا ہوں/کرتی ہوں۔			.67	
16	میں جتنا جلد ممکن ہو س خود کو پُرسکون کرنے کی کوشش کرتا ہوں۔				.81
14	میں اپنے مزاج کو قابو میں رکھتا ہوں۔				.61

Results in table 6 indicate the factor loading of items, the 25 items got loaded on five factors. On Principal component and by using the varimax rotation the factors were extracted. .35 was considered as criteria for the selection of items. So those items whose loading is equal to .35 or greater then it was selected. So by using these measures the items loading was analyzed. Five factors got emerged and with the expert opinion of scholars the last three were merged as they were depicting the same picture. 11 items got loaded in factor – I (items no. 4, 3, 7, 2, 6, 8, 5, 25, 9, 1 and 13), 8 loaded on Factor – II (Item no. 20, 17, 21, 18, 22, 19, 11 and 10) and 6 items got loaded on Factor III (item no. 15, 12, 23, 24, 16 and 14).

Table 7

Eigenvalues, Cumulative Percentage and Percentages of Variance of Variance for Three Factors of ASCIP (N = 300)

Factors	Initial Eigenvalues	% Variance	Cumulative % Variance
Factor 1	11.35	45.41	45.41
Factor 2	5.44	21.77	67.18
Factor 3	2.12	8.47	75.66

Results in the table 7 show the eigenvalues variance (percentage), which are explained by extracted factors. The Factor- I is explaining the total variance of 45.41% and eigenvalue of 11.35, which is highest values in comparison of other factors. By refereeing to the criterion, eigenvalues provide three factor solutions were deemed appropriate.

Committee approach. For the concluding decision about the items and for deciding appropriate tittles for the extracted factors the committee approach was conducted. The committee consisted of qualified and knowledgeable experts; it includes four PhD and four MPhil scholars. All of them have wide knowledge about testing and research. They did detailed analysis of all items and factors in which they fall. Then they decided the titles for the factors and these are state anger (factor – I), anger control-in (factor -II) and anger control – out (Factor-III).

Discussion. The aim of this phase of study was to construct an indigenous questionnaire for the assessment of anger among chronically ill patients. It was constructed in a manner; it measures the tendency of anger among chronically ill patients. This scale also measures the anger control among the patients along with the state anger.

There are many anger scales but after an extensive literature review (Crane, 1981; Dahlem & Deffenbacher, 2001), and critical analysis of the previously developed scales or questionnaires (Siegel, 1986; Speilberger, 1999) it was concluded that there is a need to develop an indigenous scale for assessment of anger among chronically ill patients. So for this purpose the scale was constructed in this phase.

By using a systematic approach, the scale was developed, including the empirically based anger conditions and dimensions were figured out. The FGDs were conducted to explore the details and dimensions of the anger. The FGDs were conducted with Subject Matter Experts (SME), MPhil and PhD research scholars. After conducting FGDs the committee approach was conducted in which the items were written. Then the appropriate and well-designed items were selected. The first or preliminary item-pool was generated with the help of wide empirical evicdences, furthermore the review and analysis of already developed anger scales and the insight attained from SMEs. No reverse coded items were included in the scale but as the scale was catering the three important but different aspects of anger i.e., state anger, anger control-in and anger control-out. These aspects of anger are in opposite direction with one another as for example, in case if someone is having control-in, he or she doesn't have control-out. The dimensions of the scale were determined with the help of previous literature and scales. Experts have keenly and critically looked into the details of every single statement and then they have selected 25 items out of 57 items for the scale, based on state anger and anger control. All the items were opinion statements and consisted of 4-response options i.e., very much so, moderately so, somewhat and Not at all.

The committee approach was conducted with scholars who were having extensive knowledge of research and scale construction, for having a final comment about the items of the scale. It was conducted to figure out if there is any double barrel, misleading, or ambiguous item in scale, then it should be deleted or modified. Committee was satisfied with the items and approved the items.

After the construction of the scale, for clarity of items the try out was carried out. For this purpose, 20 participants were taken and they were requested to mention if there is any difficult, ambiguity or un-clarity in any item. They haven't complained about anything and have easily completed the questionnaire. At the completion of questionnaire, the respondents were asked about it but they said they have easily done it.

After the tryout of the scale, for EFA the test was administered on the 300 chronically ill patients (cancer = 100, diabetics = 100, cardiac = 100). Then the exploratory factor analysis was computed and Principal component solution was obtained. EFA is basically a technique to figure out and classify the factors (field, 2005). Three factors were figured out, with eighenvalues greater than 1.00 were extracted. With varimax rotation the factors were computed. The three factors were extracted by taking the Kline's (1993) criteria for the item selection. Those items which have the loading of .35 and above considered for the final scale. Total five factors extracted but in the committee approach the 3, 4 and 5 factor was combined to form a one factor. So in the scale comprised of three factors. In committee approach the finalization of factors name was carried out. The committee comprised of scholars. In the committee approach the title selected for Factor-I is state anger, for factor-II the anger control-in and anger control-out for factor-III. State anger comprised of 11 items, 8 for anger control-in and 6 for anger control-out.

State anger is the name given to first factor, is derived from the literature (Etzler, Rohrmann, & Brandnt, 2014) which is associated with the present condition or situation of an individual. Like the present condition or the state changes, attitude and behavior of a person also gets change.

Anger control-in was name which is given to the second factor, is taken from the literature (Speilberger, 1988). It is about control and suppression of anger.

Anger control-out is a name given to the third factor, it is about controlling anger feelings. This name was also derived from the literature (Speilberger, 1999). This scale was constructed to measure the anger among chronically ill patients.

Phase – III: Establishment of Psychometric Properties of the Instruments

The present study was aimed to explore the most commonly reported psychological issues among chronically ill patients and to explore risk and protective factors with regard to their impact on well being and quality of life of patients.

Objective. Phase – III of the Part – I of this study was conducted to explore the psychometric properties of the all the instruments used to measure study variables. These psychometric properties include computing the alpha reliabilities of study indtruments, item-total correlation and also by computing inter-scale correlation.

Sample. The sample of the pilot study comprised of 300 chronically ill patients (cancer, diabetic and cardiac patients), taken from Oncology, general Medicine and cardiology Department of PIMS. The sample included both male and female patients. Patients having cancer, diabetes (diabetes mellitus) and cardiac patients (had experience first heart attack) were included in study. Those patients were excluded who were suffering from two or more diseases at a time, suffereing from any other disease which is not included in the present study and sufereing from any psychological illness. Table 5 explains the demographic description of the sample.

Instruments.

Personal Information Data Sheet. Personal information of the chronically ill patients includes, gender, age, family system, number of family members, duration of diagnosis, stage of disease, monthly income, education, employment status, any family member who is suffering from any chronic illness? if yes then which one and also tell the duration of that illness, symptoms of illness and distress of illness.

Anger Scale for chronically ill patients (ASCIP). In the current research this scale was developed in the Phase – I. ASCIP was constructed which comprised of 25 items scale. The scale is divided in to three dimensions (1) state anger (present state of a person that how he or she is feeling righ now), (2) anger control-out and (3) anger control-in. Items of this scale are in the form of opinion statements which has to be rated on likert scale (four point) and these are very much so, moderately so, somewhat and Not at all.

The scale helps in identifying that whether the person is experiencing the anger or have capacity or tendency to experience it. The increased score in the specific subscale indicates that the person is having a tendency to experience more anger whereas the low indicates the low tendency of having anger.

Beck Depression Inventory. It was developed by Beck and translated in Urdu (Khan, 1996), this Urdu version was administered in the current study. It's a 21 item inventory which consistent with depression criteria mentioned in DSM-IV. It is a screening tool and is not a diagnostic tool. It basically evaluates the person on 21 symptoms including failure linked with past, suicidal ideation, sadness, pessimism, worthlessness, lost of interest, loss of energy, appetite issues, sleep problems, irritability etc. BDI is used in many researches (Kuhner, Burger, Keller, & Hautzinger, 2007; Quek, Low, Razack, & Loh, 2001) and is psychometrically very sound scale. The concurrent validity (Beck, Steer & Carbin, 1988) and construct validity was established (Harris & Joyce, 2008). The Cronbach alphas of BDI mostly range from 0.75 to 0.92 (Khan, Marwat, Noor, & Fatima, 2015) and .89 (Holländare, Andersson & Engström, 2010).

Coping Strategies Questionnair (CSQ). CSQ developed by Kausar and Munir (2004) was used. It consisted of sixty-two items and as it's in Urdu language so understandable for the Pakistani people. It consisted of 4 subscales and these are active-practical coping, active-distractive coping, avoidance-focused coping and religious-focused coping. The respondent has to indicate on a 4-point scale ranging from "did not use at all" to "used quite a lot" indicating the degree to which a strategy is used. Active practical is about trying to solve the problems. Active-distractive about distracting one's mind so that he or she doesn't think about the problem. Avoidance-focused is about avoiding and considering it as tool of dealing with a problem. Religious focus is about praying and asking God for help (Kausar & Munir, 2004). This scale has four-point rating scale ranging from "did not use at all" to "use quite a lot". This scale is widely used by different researchers and was found as a psychometrically sound instrument as its alpha reliability lies from .55 to .73

(Ghazanfar & Shafiq, 2016), 0.55 to 0.78 (Kausar & Yusuf, 2011), 0.87 (Dawood & Yousaf, 2015) and 0.86 (Naveed & Yousaf, 2015).

Social Support Questionnaire. Social support was assessed by using the Social Support Questionnaire by Malik (2002). It consisted of 51 items and have five dimensions of support (informational, tangible, emotional and social network). It has four response options always, sometimes, often and never. It is highly reliable and valid indigenous scale for measuring social support. This scale is widely used in many researches and has been reported as psychometrically sound as its reliability ranges from .73 to .83 (Mushtaq & Zubair, 2015) and .94 (Manzoor, 2009).

Psychological Well Being. In the current study, for the assessment of the well-being (psychological) the Urdu translated of Ryff was used. It is translated by Ansari (2010). It consisted of 54 items and these are self-acceptance, positive relations, autonomy, environmental mastery, personal growth and purpose in life). It's a 6-point rating scale (Ansari, 2010).

Autonomy. This subscale comprised of 8 items with 5 negative stated. The score range from 8 to 40 and the high score indicate high level of autonomy. It is basically about the will power, which includes qualities like freedom, liberty and behavior regulation. Those indivuals who have autonomy have a locus of control (internal), in this case the individual doesn't need to have the endorsement or aggrement of others (Ansari, 2010).

Environmental mastery. This subscale comprised of 6 items with 2 negatively stated items assessing the sense of mastery and competence in managing the environment. It's basically about one's capability or ability to build a suitable environment which is suitable for mental and physical health of the individual. It explains the human being's ability to move in his or her life by advancing in the world and change it through physical or mental gain of any prospect. These all aspects are linked with the environmental mastery which is significant ingredient in the positive psychological functioning of an individual (Ansari, 2010).

Personal growth. This subscale comprised of 7 items with 3 negatively stated items measuring the personal development among individuals. The score range from 7 to 35. It is basically linked with the proper and complete psychological functioning personal growth is very important. There is a need to actualize one's potential and capabilities to have a personal growth. Openness is the basic and key characteristic for fully functioning person. Such an individual is continually developing excelling in his or her life (Ansari, 2010).

Positive relations with other. This subscale comprised of 6 items with 4 negatively scored items measuring trusting relationship with others. The score range from 6 to 30. Psychological well-being is also linked with establishing warm and trusting relationships with others. The ability to love is viewed as the main and central component of mental health. Self actualizers are considered to have an affectionate feelings and empathetic feelings for everyone. Other development theories also emphasized on the importance of positive relations with others and taking guidance from others, which is important for one's positive psychological development (Ansari, 2010).

Self Acceptance. This subscale comprised of 6 items measuring individual's attitude towards oneself. The score range from 6 to 30. Its characteristics include maturity, proper and optimum functioning of an individuals. Literature and theories of life span supported that for sound mental health, the individual should have his or her acceptance for past life events and above all he should be accepting his or her self. So having a positive attitude towards himself or herself for optimum functioning (Ansari, 2010).

Purpose in life. This subscale comprised of 6 items with score range from 6 to 30. For a sound mental health, it is important to have some purpose in one's life. The explanation is maturity is also linked with the having some goal of life (Ansari, 2010).

This scale is widely used scale to assessment of well-being which is a construct having varied dimensions (Ryff, 1989). The reliability estimates provided for original scale by authors for autonomy, for environmental mastery, for personal growth, for positive relations with others, for purpose in life, and for self-acceptance is .83, .86, .85, .88, .88 .91 respectively. Across different cultures it has been used for the assessment of well-being of an individual (Ansari, 2010; Kafka & Kozma, 2001). The alpha value ranges from .74 to .84 (Jibeen & Khalid, 2010) and .84 (Jibeen & Khalid, 2012).

Quality of Life Questionnaire. In the present study for the assessment of quality of life "World Health Organization Quality of Life Questionnaire" was used, which was originally developed by Power (2003) and translated into Urdu by Khalid and Kausar (2006). This version was used in current study. It basically consists of 26 items and comprised of four subscales. Subscales include functioning (physical, psychological, social relationships and environment). This questionnaire is widely used by many researchers and is psychometrically sound instrument (Ohaeri & Awadalla, 2009). The Cronbach alpha ranges from .56 to .78 (Lodhi, Raza, Montazeri, Nedjat, Yaseri, & Holakouie-Naieni, 2017) and .90 (Ilić, Šipetić-Grujičić, Grujičić, Živanović Mačužić, Kocić & Ilić, 2019).

Procedure. The data has been collected from chronically ill patients (cancer, diabetic and cardiac) both males and females, taken from General medicine, Oncology and cardiology department of PIMS. With the permission of the hospital authorities the participants were approached. With the willingness and consent of the patients the data was collected. They were explained about research aims and were ensured about the confidentiality of the information they were having the right to refuse at any point of time. Then the questionnaires (see Annexure-D) were got filled. In almost an hour the information was acquired from one patient. Patients use to take pauses (pauses of 2-3 minutes) and then reply.

Table 8

Descriptive Statistics for all Scales and their Subscales (N = 300)

Variables	α	M	SD	Score Range		Skewness	Kurtosis
				Potential	Actual		
Beck Depression Inventory							
Beck Depression Inventory	.90	13.10	10.23	0-63	3-59	2.42	1.44
Anger Scale for Chronically Ill Patients (ASCIP)							
State anger	.96	13.11	5.23	4-36	11-31	.50	.46
Anger control in	.93	20.57	6.79	4-32	8-28	.55	-1.04
Anger control out	.73	7.72	2.14	4-24	4-15	.66	.36
Social Support Questionnaire							
Social network support	.94	26.13	11.70	4-48	13-47	.54	-1.10
Esteem support	.97	23.81	12.54	4-44	11-44	.54	-1.35
Emotional support	.97	31.87	16.67	4-60	15-60	.62	-1.36
Tangible support	.90	10.97	5.60	4-20	5-20	.51	-1.34
Informational support	.90	12.95	6.16	4-24	6-24	.42	-1.25
WHO Quality Of Life Questionnaire							
Physical Functioning	.84	21.12	6.20	5-35	12-34	.41	-.83
Psychological Functioning	.74	16.88	3.34	5-30	9-25	.51	-.08
Social Dimension	.87	10.82	3.09	5-15	4-15	-.21	-1.23
Environment	.85	28.58	6.54	5-40	15-35	-.18	-.97
Perception of Quality of life and Health	.93	3.51	1.38	5-10	3-6	.41	-.85
Psychological Wellbeing Questionnaire							
Autonomy	.53	33.40	6.91	6-54	24-48	1.00	.06
Environmental mastery	.91	33.04	13.25	6-54	9-49	-.78	-.98

Personal growth	.79	33.98	11.90	6-54	9-50	-.64	-.94
Positive relations	.75	34.83	10.52	6-54	11-52	-.78	-.50
Purpose in life	.80	35.02	11.83	6-54	15-54	-.61	-1.16
Self- Acceptance	.72	31.02	9.70	6-54	16-46	.12	-1.22
Coping Strategies Questionnaire							
Active focused coping	.82	7.25	1.00	5-80	40-68	-.76	.18
Active distracting coping	.80	6.69	1.50	5-45	17-43	.02	-.67
Avoidance focused coping	.69	6.30	.68	5-120	64-99	1.56	2.12
Religious focused coping	.72	7.05	1.15	5-65	29-56	1.15	-.91

Table 8 shows that the Cronbach Alpha results indicate that most of the scales and their subscales have satisfactory reliability level. Cronbach Alpha values ranges from .53 to .97 which indicates that all instruments are having sound psychometric properties. The benchmark for alpha reliability value is explained as it should be higher than 0.5 (Ali, 2018). The alpha coefficient of Beck Depression Inventory is .90, which is in satisfactory range. The alpha reliability of ASCIP ranges from .73 to .96, the social support questionnaire reliability values ranges from .90 to .97, for WHO Quality of life it ranges from .74 to .93 and for coping strategies questionnaire it's .69 to .82, these all values fall within the satisfactory range of reliabilities. For psychological well-being scale the alpha reliabilities ranges from .53 to .91. Only autonomy is having reliability of .53 which is not that much high, other than this all the subscales have satisfactorily high values of reliability. The benchmark for alpha reliability value is explained as it should be higher than 0.5 (Ali, 2018). Furthermore, skwness and kurtosis values fall within the acceptable range of +2 to -2 (George & Mallery, 2010).

Table 9

Item-total Correlation of Beck Depression Inventory (N = 300)

Item. No	r	Item. No	r	Item. No	r
1.	.67**	9.	.84**	17.	.37**
2.	.65**	10.	.69**	18.	.45**
3.	.77**	11.	.64**	19.	.72**
4.	.33**	12.	.93**	20.	.31**
5.	.87**	13.	.88**	21.	.22**
6.	.60**	14.	.79**		
7.	.85**	15.	.51**		
8.	.91**	16.	.35**		

Results in the Table 9 indicate that the magnitude of relationship of all the items with total score ranging from .22 to .93. The recommended level of item total correlation is greater than 0.2 (Hisham et al., 2018; Streiner, Norman & Cairney, 1995).

Table 10

Item-total Correlation of State Anger, anger control-in and anger control-out of ASCIP (N = 300)

State Anger				Anger Control-In		Anger Control-Out	
Item. No	r	Item. No	r	Item. No	r	Item. No	r
2.	.79**	15.	.82**	16.	.64**	21.	.81**
4.	.96**	22.	.72**	18.	.77**	26.	.39**
6.	.96**	57.	.90**	36.	.87**	30.	.81**
8.	.96**			38.	.86**	32.	.41**
10.	.95**			40.	.80**	53.	.81**
11.	.95**			44.	.92**	54.	.59**
12.	.98**			46.	.88**		
14.	.95**			48.	.88**		

Results in the Table 10 indicate that the magnitude of relationship of all the items with total score ranging from .39 to .98. The recommended level of item total correlation is greater than 0.2 (Hisham et al., 2018; Streiner, Norman & Cairney, 1995).

Table 11

Item-total Correlation of Informational, tangible, emotional, esteem and social networking Support of Social Support Questionnaire Scale (N = 300)

Informational Support		Tangible Support		Emotional Support		Esteem Support		Social Network Support	
Item. No	r	Item. No	r	Item. No	r	Item. No	r	Item. No	r
5.	$.84^{**}$	4.	$.56^{**}$	2.	$.47^{**}$	3.	$.96^{**}$	1.	$.12^{*}$
10.	$.95^{**}$	9.	$.81^{**}$	7.	$.72^{**}$	8.	$.88^{**}$	6.	$.71^{**}$
16.	$.52^{**}$	31.	$.96^{**}$	12.	$.98^{**}$	13.	$.77^{**}$	11.	$.91^{**}$
28.	$.92^{**}$	40.	$.94^{**}$	15.	$.78^{**}$	19.	$.84^{**}$	14.	$.91^{**}$
36.	$.88^{**}$	49.	$.97^{**}$	20.	$.95^{**}$	22.	$.96^{**}$	18.	$.91^{**}$
40.	$.86^{**}$			26.	$.75^{**}$	25.	$.84^{**}$	21.	$.66^{**}$
				29.	$.97^{**}$	32.	$.93^{**}$	24.	$.82^{**}$
				35.	$.96^{**}$	34.	$.80^{**}$	27.	$.74^{**}$
				38.	$.95^{**}$	37.	$.96^{**}$	30.	$.92^{**}$
				41.	$.61^{**}$	42.	$.96^{**}$	33.	$.91^{**}$
				43.	$.98^{**}$	45.	$.92^{**}$	39.	$.89^{**}$
				46.	$.96^{**}$			50.	$.85^{**}$
				48.	$.94^{**}$				
				51.	$.94^{**}$				

Results in the Table 11 indicate that the magnitude of relationship of all the items with total score ranging from .12 to .98. The recommended level of item total correlation is greater than 0.2 (Hisham et al., 2018; Streiner, Norman & Cairney, 1995).

Table 12

Item-total Correlation of Physical Functioning, psychological functioning, social relationships, environment and perception of quality of life of WHO Quality of life Questionnaire (N = 300)

Physical functioning		Psychological functioning		Social Relationships		Environment		Perception of quality of life	
Item. No	r	Item. No	r	Item. No	r	Item. No	r	Item. No	r
3.	.60**	5.	.61**	19.	.92**	8.	.88**	1.	.97**
4.	.64**	6.	.40**	20.	.77**	9.	.90**	2.	.96**
10.	.66**	7.	.73**	21.	.91**	12.	.52**		
15.	.40**	11.	.72**			13.	.91**		
16.	.89**	18.	.77**			14.	.91**		
17.	.84**	26.	.68**			22.	.90**		
25.	.82**					23.	.17**		
						24.	.90**		

Results in the Table 12 indicate that the magnitude of relationship of all the items with total score ranging from .40 to .97. The recommended level of item total correlation is greater than 0.2 (Hisham et al., 2018; Streiner, Norman & Cairney, 1995).

Table 13

Item-total Correlation of Environmental Mastery, self-acceptance, positive relations with others, autonomy, purpose in life and personal growth of Psychological Well-Being Questionnaire (N = 300)

Environmental Mastery		Self-Acceptance		Positive Relations with others		Autonomy		Purpose in Life		Personal Growth	
Item. No	r	Item. No	r	Item. No	r	Item. No	r	Item. No	r	Item. No	r
2.	.91**	6.	.14**	1.	.89**	9.	.58**	8.	.39**	3.	.15**
7.	.93**	15.	.82**	5.	.29**	13.	.39**	12.	.41**	17.	.83**
11.	.73**	18.	.43**	10.	.19*	22.	.65**	21.	.38**	20.	.86**
16.	.17**	24.	.36**	14.	.42**	27.	.66**	26.	.70**	25.	.87**
19.	.93**	34.	.71**	23.	.90**	30.	.26**	29.	.91**	32.	.87**
28.	.54**	39.	.29**	31.	.55**	42.	.20*	32.	.84**	40.	.23**
35.	.95**	43.	.60**	33.	.76**	48.	.33**	37.	.80**	45.	.84**

49.	.72**	44.	.60**	38.	.91**	51.	.47**	41.	.90**	50.	.90**
53.	.92**	52.	.81**	47.	.90**			46.	.28**	54.	.45**

Results in the Table 13 indicate that the magnitude of relationship of all the items with total score ranging from .14 to .95. The recommended level of item total correlation is greater than 0.2 (Hisham et al., 2018; Streiner, Norman & Cairney, 1995).

Table 14

Item-total Correlation of active Focused, active distracting, avoidance-focused and religious Coping Strategies of Coping Strategies Questionnaire (N = 300)

Active Focused Coping Strategies		Active Distracting Coping Strategies		Avoidance - Focused Coping Strategies				Religious - Focused Coping Strategies	
Item. No	r	Item. No	r	Item. No	r	Item. No	r	Item. No	r
3.	.97**	7.	.79**	1.	.58**	36.	.12*	2.	.70**
5.	.62**	8.	.22**	4.	.39**	38.	.14**	6.	.60**
23.	.61**	13.	.62**	10.	.62**	44.	.48**	9.	.14*
29.	.44**	14.	.94**	11.	.35**	45.	.74**	15.	.82**
39.	.86**	17.	.25**	12.	.18**	46.	.25**	19.	.49**
41.	.30**	21.	.81**	16.	.56**	47.	.22**	25.	.64**
42.	.34**	35.	.80**	18.	.61**	50.	.72**	32.	.67**
52.	.17**	43.	.81**	20.	.60**	56.	.73**	34.	.65**
54.	.26**	49.	.16**	22.	.71**			37.	.78**
55.	.66**			24.	.64**			40.	.12*
57.	.78**			26.	.10*			48.	.60**
58.	.78**			27.	.10*			51.	.23**
59.	.53**			28.	.28**			53.	.56**
60.	.45**			30.	.10*				
61.	.56**			31.	.11*				
62.	.13*			33.	.20**				

Results in the Table 14 indicate that the magnitude of relationship of all the items with total score ranging from .10 to .97. The recommended level of item total correlation is greater than 0.2 (Hisham et al., 2018; Streiner, Norman & Cairney, 1995).

Table 15

Correlation of ASCIP, Beck Depression Inventory, Coping Strategies Questionnaire, Social Support Questionnaire, Psychological well-being Questionnaire and Quality of Life Questionnaire of chronically patients and diabetic Patients (n=300, 100)

	1	2	3	4	5	6	7	8	9	10	11	12	13	14	15	16	17	18	19	20	21	22	23	24
1	-	.32**	.12*	.13*	-.31**	-.12*	-.11*	-.22**	.36**	.42**	.37**	.39**	.34**	-.28**	-.11*	-.34**	.12*	-.26**	-.32**	-.09	-.24**	-.20**	-.19**	.21**
2	.82**	-	-.14**	.56**	-.57**	-.17**	.11*	.04	.03	.21**	.14**	.19**	.10*	.13*	.07	-.01	-.13*	.07	.01	-.09	-.30**	-.33**	-.20**	.47**
3	.18*	-.21*	-	-.09	-.15**	-.02	-.47**	-.38**	.14**	-.04	-.05	-.07	-.01	-.11*	20**	-.12*	-.08	.05	-.04	-.05	-.12*	-.22**	-.27**	-.06
4	.52**	.68**	-.17*	-	-.31**	-.11*	.07	.05	-.15**	-.05	-.10*	-.05	-.08	.22**	.15**	.17**	-.10*	.21**	.21**	-.07	-.10*	-.16**	-.08	.15**
5	-.87**	-.79**	-.03	-.57**	-	.35**	.13*	.46**	-.06	-.12*	-.07	-.10*	-.08	-.15**	-.33**	-.02	.08	-.04	-.10*	.30**	.43**	.74**	.64**	-.28**
6	-.30**	-.30**	.11	-.35**	.49**	-	.40**	.23**	.14**	-.06	-.06	-.08	-.07	.09	-.13*	.21**	.03	.06	.10*	.72**	.05	.23**	.44**	-.01
7	.14	.31**	-.53**	.16	-.18*	.22*	-	.32**	-.09	.05	-.02	.01	-.02	.12*	-.29**	.15**	-.05	.10*	.08	.47**	.14**	.25**	.40**	.20**
8	-.42**	.09	-.44**	.06	.40**	.18*	.03	-	-.19**	-.00	.01	.01	.01	.03	-.11*	.03	-.02	.07	-.06	.09	.08	.48**	.51**	-.00
9	.44**	.21*	.21*	.13	-.32**	.22*	.05	-.50**	-	.83**	.86**	.82**	.80**	-.80**	-.59**	-.77**	.53**	-.83**	-.76**	.12*	-.18**	.02	.06	.03
10	.87**	.82**	-.19*	.54**	-.87**	-.35**	.44**	-.32**	.23**	-	.97**	.98**	.92**	-.84**	-.57**	-.85**	.55**	-.82**	-.84**	-.11*	-.28**	-.00	-.03	.17**
11	.75**	.88**	-.38**	.61**	-.77**	-.32**	.42**	-.03	.23*	.91**	-	.99**	.95**	-.88**	-.64**	-.86**	.65**	-.91**	-.86**	-.11*	-.29**	.01	-.01	.09
12	.72**	.84**	-.38**	.61**	-.80**	-.32**	.40**	-.04	.16	.90**	.95**	-	.96**	-.87**	-.62**	-.83**	.66**	-.87**	-.83**	-.15**	-.30**	-.00	-.05	.13*
13	.45**	.53**	-.20*	.43**	-.66**	-.33**	.23*	-.13	.13	.68**	.78**	.80**	-	-.89**	-.58**	-.81**	.73**	-.84**	-.79**	-.13*	-.33**	-.00	-.10*	.06
14	.17*	.46**	-.61**	.13	-.09	-.04	.24**	.44**	-.01	.28**	.44**	.34**	.05	-	.68**	.92**	-.64**	.87**	.89**	.08	.08	-.22**	-.06	.09
15	.09	-.07	.25**	-.17*	-.21*	-.27**	-.51**	-.08	-.11	.00	-.07	-.06	.09	.07	-	.53**	-.40**	.68**	.57**	-.23**	-.22**	-.35**	-.40**	-.13*
16	-.43**	-.20*	-.48**	-.18*	.49**	.24**	.04	.46**	-.14	-.23*	-.01	.01	.05	.29**	-.34**	-	-.42**	.82**	.94**	.15**	.11*	-.12*	.02	-.02
17	-.42**	-.31**	-.30**	-.18*	.28**	-.07	-.28**	.20*	-.23*	-.25**	-.04	-.02	.31**	.01	.26**	.48**	-	-.66**	-.44**	-.04	-.27**	.13*	.03	-.26**
18	.19*	.12	.26**	.05	-.09	.03	-.00	.00	-.09	.10	.02	.04	-.03	-.23*	.10	-.06	-.10	-	.86**	.10	.15**	-.10*	-.05	.08
19	-.19*	-.11	-.16	.06	.15	.01	-.03	.04	.02	-.07	.07	.12	.30**	-.25**	-.32**	.55**	.52**	.42**	-	.07	.06	-.25**	-.13*	-.06
20	-.11	-.21*	.03	-.32**	.35**	.72**	.30**	-.09	.39**	-.24**	-.27**	-.33**	-.49**	.15	-.30**	.06	-.31**	.02	-.13	-	.34**	.43**	.65**	.13*
21	-.42**	-.45**	-.10	-.24**	.46**	.19*	.01	-.06	-.03	-.49**	-.58**	-.52**	-.73**	-.12	-.33**	.02	-.20*	-.13	-.09	.42**	-	.64**	.64**	-.14**
22	-.74**	-.59**	-.18*	-.49**	.79**	.34**	-.09	.45**	-.31**	-.77**	-.73**	-.75**	-.83**	.16	-.04	.25**	.02	-.08	-.17*	.38**	.63**	-	.87**	-.24**
23	-.48**	-.31**	-.26**	-.32**	.64**	.43**	.13	.45**	-.17*	-.54**	-.51**	-.55**	-.85**	.31**	-.27**	.19*	-.24**	-.05	-.25**	.60**	.67**	.87**	-	-.10
24	.76**	.72**	-.11	.41**	-.46**	.00	.30**	-.05	.27**	.72**	.71**	.63**	.27**	.44**	-.26**	.03	-.35**	.08	-.13	.10	-.28**	-.47**	-.12	-

Note. The values above the diagonal show correlation coefficient for all chronically ill patients andbelow the diagonal show correlation for the diabetic patients.

1.Beck Depression Inventory, 2. State Anger, 3.Anger Control-in 4.Anger Control-Out. 5. Active–Focused Coping Strategies 6. Distracting–Focused Coping Strategies 7. Avoidance Focused Coping Strategies. 8. Religious–Focused Coping Strategies. 9 Informational Support. 10. Tangible Support. 11. Emotional Support. 12. Esteem Support. 13. Social Network Support. 14. Environmental Mastery. 15. Self-Acceptance. 16. Positive relations with others. 17. Autonomy. 18. Purpose in life. 19. Personal Growth. 20. Physical functioning. 21. Psychological Functioning. 22. Social relationships 23. Environment. 24. Perception of quality of life and health.

Table 15 indicates that there is a significant positive relationship of depression with state anger, anger control-in, anger control-out, informational support, tangible support, emotional support, esteem support, social network support and autonomy among chronically ill patients. It also indicates that there is a significant negative relationship between coping strategies (active focused, religious focused, avoidance focused), self-acceptance, environmental mastery, purpose in life, personal growth, positive relations with others, functioning (physical, psychological) social relations and environment. Results indicates that there is a positive relationship of state anger with depression, anger control-in, anger control-out, avoidance focused coping, tangible support, emotional support, esteem support, social network support and environmental mastery whereas there is significant negative relationship of state anger with active focused coping, active distracting coping, autonomy, psychological functioning, social relationships and environment. Anger control-in is significantly positively associated with informational support and self-acceptance whereas it is negatively correlated with active focused-coping strategies, avoidance focused coping strategies, religious focused coping strategies, environmental mastery, positive relations with others, psychological functioning, social relations and environment. Anger control – out is negatively correlated with active focused coping active distracting coping, informational support, emotional support, autonomy, psychological functioning and social relations with others whereas anger control – out is positively correlated with environmental mastery, personal growth and autonomy among chronically ill patients.

Results revealed that depression is significantly positively correlated with state anger, anger control-in, anger control-out, informational support, tangible support, esteem support, social network support and purpose in life whereas it is negatively correlated with active focused coping strategies, active distracting coping strategies, religious focused coping strategies, positive relations with others, autonomy, personal growth, psychological functioning, social relations with others and environment among diabetic patients. State anger is significantly positively correlated with depression, anger control – out, avoidance focused coping strategies, informational support, tangible support, esteem support, social network support and environmental mastery, whereas it (state anger) is significantly negatively anger control- in, active focused coping strategies, active distractive coping strategies , positive relations with others, autonomy, physical functioning, psychological functioning, social relationships and environment among diabetic patients. Anger control-in is negatively associated with state anger, anger control-out, avoidance focused coping strategies, religious focused coping strategies, tangible support, esteem support, social network support, environmental mastery, positive relations with others, autonomy, social relationships and environment, whereas it (anger control-in) is positively associated with depression, informational support, self-acceptance and purpose in life among diabetic patients. Anger control- out is negatively associated with active focused coping strategies, active distracting coping strategies, self-acceptance, positive relations with others, autonomy, physical functioning, psychological functioning, social relationships and environment among diabetic patients.

Table 16

Correlation of ASCIP, Beck Depression Inventory, Coping Strategies Questionnaire, Social Support Questionnaire, Psychological well-being Questionnaire and Quality of Life Questionnaire of cancer and cardiac Patients (n=100, 100)

	1	2	3	4	5	6	7	8	9	10	11	12	13	14	15	16	17	18	19	20	21	22	23	24
1	1	.74**	.45**	.43**	-.83**	-.06	-.30**	-.58**	.57**	.70**	.59**	.55**	.31**	.26**	.36**	-.38**	-.12	.25**	-.06	.07	-.29**	-.67**	-.45**	.54**
2	.06	1	-.07	.62**	-.73**	-.15	.02	.02	.20*	.80**	.82**	.80**	.40**	.67**	.15	-.04	-.01	.26**	.12	-.07	-.34**	-.45**	-.24**	.63**
3	-.01	-.15	1	-.08	-.40**	-.05	-.67**	-.64**	.41**	-.12	-.24**	-.22*	.03	-.57**	.52**	-.48**	-.12	.40**	.06	-.03	-.19*	-.47**	-.52**	-.15
4	.08	.48**	-.05	1	-.52**	-.26**	-.05	.03	-.01	.49**	.49**	.52**	.30**	.32**	.21*	-.19*	.14	.14	.06	-.25**	-.26**	-.30**	-.23*	.26**
5	.04	-.13	-.03	.01	1	.36**	.32**	.51**	-.32**	-.69**	-.60**	-.65**	-.52**	-.15	-.62**	.42**	-.13	-.35**	-.17*	.35**	.34**	.75**	.69**	-.23**
6	-.06	-.07	-.08	.11	.21*	1	.42**	.09	.33**	.07	.10	.04	.04	.13	-.26**	.45**	-.09	.05	-.05	.77**	-.21*	.02	.22*	.42**
7	-.06	.06	-.08	.11	.20*	.64**	1	.35**	-.07	.30**	.32**	.28**	.07	.46**	-.47**	.50**	.05	-.14	-.03	.43**	-.01	.33**	.41**	.37**
8	-.07	.01	-.08	.05	.50**	.51**	.75**	1	-.63**	-.17*	.03	.04	-.04	.31**	-.30**	.55**	.16	.07	.15	-.04	-.09	.45**	.43**	.04
9	-.11	-.20*	-.02	.02	.39**	.83**	.27**	.24**	1	.20*	.19*	.05	-.00	.02	.02	-.25**	-.20*	-.05	-.05	.54**	-.10	-.30**	-.08	.33**
10	-.04	-.20*	-.04	-.00	.87**	.55**	.35**	.57**	.69**	1	.92**	.93**	.60**	.60**	.22*	.09	.15	.20*	.12	.03	-.44**	-.57**	-.37**	.70**
11	-.13	-.25**	.01	-.04	.59**	.56**	.18*	.16	.85**	.83**	1	.95**	.73**	.67**	.18*	.20*	.35**	.19*	.33**	.04	-.58**	-.60**	-.37**	.65**
12	-.04	-.22*	.02	-.01	.75**	.40**	.17*	.14	.72**	.82**	.91**	1	.74**	.59**	.24**	.22*	.34**	.18*	.37**	-.11	-.52**	-.60**	-.45**	.60**
13	-.09	-.13	-.01	.04	.57**	.44**	.44**	.27**	.61**	.61**	.74**	.80**	1	.16	.52**	.19*	.67**	.31**	.67**	-.26**	-.76**	-.81**	-.80**	.11
14	.03	.08	-.01	.01	-.73**	-.12	-.42**	-.29**	-.26**	-.60**	-.56**	-.75**	-.80**	1	-.29**	.41**	-.14	-.07	-.04	.21*	-.08	.04	.27**	.63**
15	.09	.11	-.06	-.02	-.42**	-.32**	-.38**	-.10	-.52**	-.40**	-.61**	-.72**	-.92**	.79**	1	-.42**	.50**	.58**	.20*	-.44**	-.49**	-.65**	-.76**	-.22*
16	.06	.02	-.01	.09	-.63**	.26**	-.23*	-.52**	.26**	-.41**	-.08	-.17*	-.17*	.58**	.07	1	.01	-.09	.44**	.20*	-.16	.16	.20*	.29**
17	-.02	-.10	.01	.06	.08	.41**	.24**	-.25**	.56**	.24**	.60**	.67**	.65**	-.46**	-.71**	.40**	1	.10	.56**	-.28**	-.59**	-.45**	-.50**	-.17
18	.11	.15	-.02	.03	.09	-.41**	.04	.38**	-.64**	-.20*	-.66**	-.54**	-.43**	.14	.42**	-.47**	-.81**	1	.19*	-.06	-.48**	-.36**	-.38**	.06
19	.02	.10	-.03	.09	-.75**	.09	-.41**	-.55**	.06	-.57**	-.27**	-.45**	-.44**	.81**	.38**	.88**	.04	-.32**	1	-.25**	-.54**	-.49**	-.54**	-.05
20	-.07	.02	-.11	.14	.18*	.65**	.76**	.39**	.45**	.36**	.45**	.35**	.72**	-.50**	-.58**	-.06	.49**	-.33**	-.20*	1	-.00	.17*	.48**	.51**
21	-.07	-.07	-.04	.03	.61**	.33**	.61**	.55**	.30**	.57**	.48**	.48**	.79**	-.78**	-.67**	-.57**	.16	.07	-.68**	.75**	1	.67**	.58**	-.25**
22	.02	-.05	-.08	.10	.74**	.37**	.65**	.55**	.34**	.71**	.55**	.68**	.81**	-.87**	-.66**	-.50**	.40**	-.04	-.74**	.71**	.86**	1	.89**	-.19*
23	-.05	-.07	-.09	.12	.61**	.75**	.76**	.64**	.67**	.75**	.68**	.67**	.84**	-.67**	-.67**	-.22*	.47**	-.24**	-.46**	.84**	.81**	.88**	1	.15
24	-.07	.04	.08	-.10	-.11	-.60**	-.17*	.00	-.52**	-.39**	-.44**	-.35**	.02	-.03	-.11	-.27**	-.41**	.53**	-.18*	-.21*	.18*	-.08	-.27**	1

Note: The values above the diagonal show correlation coefficient for all cancer patients and cardiac patients below the diagonal.

1.Beck Depression Inventory, 2. State Anger, 3.Anger Control-in 4.Anger Control-Out. 5. Active–Focused Coping Strategies 6. Distracting–Focused Coping Strategies 7. Avoidance Focused Coping Strategies. 8. Religious–Focused Coping Strategies. 9 Informational Support. 10. Tangible Support. 11. Emotional Support. 12. Esteem Support. 13. Social Network Support. 14. Environmental Mastery. 15. Self-Acceptance. 16. Positive relations with others. 17. Autonomy. 18. Purpose in life. 19. Personal Growth. 20. Physical functioning. 21. Psychological Functioning. 22. Social relationships 23. Environment. 24. Perception of quality of life and health.

Table 16 indicates that there is significant positive relationship of depression with state anger, anger control-in, anger control-out, informational support, tangible support, emotional support, esteem support, social network support, environmental mastery, self-acceptance and purpose in life whereas it (depression) is negatively correlated with active focused-coping strategies, avoidance focused coping strategies, religious focused coping strategies, psychological functioning, social relationships and environment among cancer patients. State anger is positively correlated with anger control-out, informational support, tangible support, emotional support, esteem support, social network support, environmental mastery and purpose in life whereas it is negatively correlated with active focused-coping strategies, psychological functioning, social relationships and environment among cancer patients. Anger control-in is positively correlated with informational support, self-acceptance and purpose in life, where as it is negatively correlated with

Results indicates that that there is significant positive relationship of state anger with anger control-out whereas state anger is negatively correlated with anger control-out, informational support, tangible support and esteem support among cardiac patients.

Discussion. The present study was conducted to explore the most commonly reported psychological issues among chronically ill patients. Furthermore, it also deals with the exploration of risk and protective factors for quality of life and psychological well-being. For this purposes first of all the psychological issues, risk and protective factors, which are related to chronic illness, were explored. For this purpose, focus group discussion and interviews were conducted in order to explore the psychological issues, risk and protective factors. Then after the exploration and identification they were enlisted as depression, anger (psychological issues), social support and coping strategies (risk and protective factors).

This section of the study was conducted to explore the psychometric properties of the instruments. The main objective was to check the psychometric suitability of the instruments. Beck Depression Inventory (Khan, 1996) was selected to assess the depression among patients, Social Support Scale (Malik, 2002) for the assessment of social support, Coping Strategies Questionnaire (Kausar & Munir,

2004) for the assessment of coping strategies, WHO Quality of Life Questionnaire by Khalid and Kausar (2006) for the assessment of quality of life, Psychological wellbeing(Ansari, 2010) was used for the assessment of psychological well-being and for the assessment of anger among chronically ill patients the ASCIP was developed in the previous phase of the study. The instruments were administered on 300 chronically ill patients. They were taken from the oncology, general medicine and cardiac departments of PIMS hospital. The reliability of the scales and subscales were established, which indicates that instruments are psychometrically sound. The Cronbach Alpha results indicate that most of the scales and their subscales have satisfactory reliability level. Cronbach Alpha values ranges from .53 to .96 and the item-total correlation also indicated that the magnitude is within the considerable range, which indicates that all instruments are having sound psychometric properties.

For the assessment of depression, Beck Depression Inventory (Khan, 1996) was used. The item-total correlation was computed and the results of indicated that the magnitude is within the considerable range, so the instrument is psychometrically sound. The alpha reliability was .90 which is psychometrically very sound (Frank-Stromborg & Oslen, 2004). BDI is used in many researches (Kuhner, Burger, Keller, & Hautzinger, 2007; Quek, Low, Razack, & Loh, 2001) and is psychometrically very sound scale. The Cronbach alphas of BDI mostly range from 0.75 to 0.92 (Khan, Marwat, Noor, & Fatima, 2015).

For the assessment of anger, the ASCIP was used and the alpha reliability of the subscales ranges from .73 to .96 which is a good reliability (Frank-Stromborg, & Oslen, 2004). The item-total correlation was computed and the results of indicated that the magnitude is within the considerable range, so the instrument is psychometrically sound.

Coping strategies were assessed through the CSQ by Kausar and Munir (2004). The questionnaire assesses four types of copings namely as active-practical, active-distractive, avoidance-focused and religious-focused. It has been used in many researches and is psychologically very sound instrument for the present research its alpha reliability ranges from .69 to .82 which is a good reliability (Frank-Stromborg & Oslen, 2004). Ghazanfar and Shafiq reported that the reliability of CSQ lies from .55 to .73 (Ghazanfar & Shafiq, 2016). The item-total correlation was computed and the results of indicated that the magnitude is within the considerable range, so the instrument is psychometrically sound.

For the assessment of the social support, Social Support Scale (Malik, 2002) was used. The item-total correlation was computed and the results of indicated that the magnitude is within the considerable range, so the instrument is psychometrically sound. It has been used in many researches it is psychometrically very sound scale (Negovan, 2010) and its reliability ranges from .73 to .83 (Mushtaq & Zubair, 2015). In the present research the alpha reliability for its subscales ranges from .90 to .93.

Psychological wellbeing is assessed by using Psychological well-being (Ansari, 2010). It was used in many researchers (Negovan, 2010) and its psychometrically very sound instrument. The item-total correlation was computed and the results of indicated that the magnitude is within the considerable range, so the instrument is psychometrically sound. In the present research its reliability ranges from .53 to .91 which falls in the category of good, only autonomy is having reliability of .53 which is not that much high, other than this all the subscales have satisfactorily high values of reliability.

In the present research the quality of life of the chronically ill patients was assessed through WHO Quality of Life Questionnaire by Khalid and Kausar (2006) in the present research the alpha reliability of this questionnaire ranges from .74 to .93, which is satisfactory in range. The item-total correlation was computed and the results of indicated that all the items are significantly correlated with the total score of the respective sub-scale. This questionnaire is widely used by many researchers and is psychometrically sound instrument (Ohaeri & Awadalla, 2009).

All the instruments used in present study have reliability of .6 and above which indicates that the instruments were internally consistent (Nunnally& Bernstein, 1994). The item-total coorelation was computed in the main study data to further explore the range of magnitude values.

Furthermore, it was also indicated by the results that all other values are within the normal range and data values fall within normal distribution (Field, 2005). Results of skewness and kurtosis indicate that the values are within normal range of +2 to -2, which indicates that, the values of skewness and kurtosis of all the instruments was not problematic (Muthen & Kaplan, 1985). Data was normally distributed.

Chapter - IV

Part - II

Present study was conducted to explore the psychological issues among chronically ill patients and it also aimed to explore risk and protective factors for psychological well-being and quality of life. Part –II of the present study deals with main study.

Objectives

Main study was conducted to achieve following objectives.

1. To find out the level of psychological issues (anger and depression) among chronically ill patients (including Cardiac, cancer, and diabetes patients).

2. To find out impact of psychological issues on well being and quality of life of chronically ill patients (including Cardiac, cancer, and diabetes patients).

3. To find out the moderating role of risk and protectitve in relationship of psychological issues (anger and depression) with psychological wellbeing and quality of life among chronically ill patients (including Cardiac, cancer, and diabetes patients).

4. To find out the effects of demographic, social and familial variables (i.e., gender, family history, family system, education, marital status, disease status and stage).

Hypotheses

Following hypotheses were formulated for present study:

1. There is a negative relationship of depression with quality of life and psychological well-being of chronically ill patients (cardiac, cancer and diabetics).

2. There is a negative relationship of anger with quality of life and psychological well-being of chronically ill patients (cardiac, cancer and diabetics).

3. Depression negatively predicts the quality of life and psychological well-being of chronically ill patients (cardiac, cancer and diabetics).

4.   Anger negatively predicts the quality of life and psychological well-being of chronically ill patients (cardiac, cancer and diabetics).

5.   Risk and protective factors (social support and coping) act as a moderator in relationship between the psychological issues and quality of life and psychological well-being among chronically ill patients (cardiac, cancer and diabetics).

Instruments

The instruments used in the main study are.

1.   Beck Depression Inventory (Khan, 1996)

2.   ASCIP (Developed in present study Phase –II of Part –I)

3.   Coping Strategies Questionnaire (Kausar & Munir, 2004).

4.   Social Support Scale (Malik, 2002).

5.   Psychological well being (Ansari, 2010).

6.   WHO Quality of Life Questionnaire (Khalid & Kausar, 2006)

Note: Details of instruments are in the instrument section of Phase – III (establishment of psychometric properties of the instruments).

Sample

The sample of the main study comprised of 500 chronically ill patients (cardiac, cancer and diabetic patients), taken from Oncology, Cardiac and General Medicine Department of PIMS. Sample comprised of 131 males and 369 females, 350 were married and 150 unmarried, 284 are from the nuclear family system and 214 were from joint family system.

Inclusion criteria. Patients having heart diseases, cancer and diabetes were included. Cardiac patients were those who have experienced only one heart attack and have only this problem.

Exclusion criteria. Patients having more than two illnesses at a time, suffering from any psychological disorder along with the chronic diseases or suffering from the chronic disease other than these diseases were not include in the study.

Table 17

Descriptive Characteristics of the Sample (N=500)

Variables	f	%	M	SD
Disease				
Diabetes	104	20.8		
Cancer	196	39.2		
Cardiac	200	40.0		
Duration of illness			13.25	12.28
Stage of disease				
Stage 4 (cancer)	196	39.2		
First heart attack (cardiac)	200	40.0		
Insulin dependent (diabetes)	104	20.8		
Gender				
Male	131	26.2		
Female	369	73.8		
Age			32.81	13.66
Education				
Un educated	155	31.0		
Primary	58	11.6		
Middle	37	7.4		
Matric	118	23.6		
FA/F.Sc	71	14.2		
BA/B.Sc	57	11.4		
M.Sc	4	.8		
Marital Status				
Married	350	70.0		
Unmarried	150	30.0		
Family system				
Nuclear	286	57.2		
Joint	214	42.8		
Employment Status				
Employed	102	20.4		
Unemployed	398	79.6		
Monthly Income				
Less than 10000	253	50.6		

Between 10000–50000	224	44.8
Above 50000	23	4.6
Number of family members		
1-5 members	242	48.4
6-10 members	181	36.2
11-15 members	77	15.4

Table 17 shows the demographic description of the sample. The main study comprised of 500 chronically ill patients.

Procedure

For the main study the information was collected from the chronically ill patients (cancer, cardiac and diabetic) both males and females, taken from PIMS, hospital. With the permission of authorities, the patients were approached. Patients were explained about the research and with their consent the instruments were got filled by them. It took almost an hour to get information from one patient. Patients use to take pauses (pauses of 2-3 minutes) and then reply, that's why the data was not collected in one session. They were also provided with the counseling even after the completion of data collection. The APA ethical guidelines were followed while handling with participants. As many patients need counseling so the counseling sessions were provided to them. The follow-up sessions were taken and patients have also shown improvement in their psychological symptoms.

Chapter V

RESULTS

Present study was conducted to explore the psychological issues among chronically ill patients and it also aimed to explore risk and protective factors for psychological well-being and quality of life.

Table 18

Descriptive Statistics for all Scales and their Subscales (N = 500)

Variables	α	M	SD	Score Range Potential	Actual	Skewness	Kurtosis
				Beck Depression Inventory			
Beck Depression Inventory	.94	15.36	13.83	0-63	3-59	2.04	.76
				ASCIP			
State anger	.96	12.92	4.96	4-36	11-31	2.67	.37
Anger control in	.94	20.57	6.83	4-32	8-28	-.56	-1.04
Anger control out	.74	7.50	2.71	4-24	4-14	.39	-1.18
				Social Support Questionnaire			
Social network support	.76	41.8	5.37	4-48	24-47	-.49	-1.13
Esteem support	.87	39.78	5.09	4-44	22-44	-1.40	1.16
Emotional support	.82	54.27	5.35	4-60	23-60	-1.67	3.96
Tangible support	.74	16.98	3.61	4-20	5-20	-1.60	2.33
Informational support	.63	18.99	3.79	4-24	6-24	-.70	.20
				WHO Quality Of Life Questionnaire			
Physical Functioning	.79	77.10	26.53	5-35	7-31	.19	-.70
Psychological Functioning	.71	65.78	14.82	5-30	5-25	-.57	1.45
Social Relationships	.91	41.05	14.95	5-15	3-15	-.17	-1.28
Environment	.82	114.99	28.31	5-40	15-40	.24	-1.28
Perception of Quality of life and Health	.90	13.81	5.34	5-10	2-6	.49	-.70

Continued...

Variables	α	M	SD	Score Range		Skewness	Kurtosis
				Potential	Actual		
Psychological Wellbeing Questionnaire							
Autonomy	.71	34.01	11.11	6-54	19-54	.48	-.62
Environmental mastery	.93	31.53	14.16	6-54	9-49	-.50	-1.42
Personal growth	.72	30.53	10.81	6-54	9-46	-.43	-.10
Positive relations	.76	33.52	11.09	6-54	11-52	-.50	-.89
Purpose in life	.73	31.07	10.64	6-54	15-49	-.31	-1.41
Self- Acceptance	.80	33.46	11.52	6-54	16-51	-.02	-1.23
Coping Strategies Questionnaire							
Active focused coping	.82	58.24	7.76	5-80	40-68	-.77	.36
Active distracting coping	.77	29.50	5.86	5-45	19-39	.53	-1.11
Avoidance focused coping	.71	76.18	8.05	5-120	67-104	1.86	4.31
Religious focused coping	.80	45.15	7.84	5-65	27-54	-.64	-.81

Table 18 shows the mean, standard deviation, score range (minimum and maximum), kurtosis and skewness. The Cronbach Alpha values ranges from .63 to .96 which indicates that the instruments are psychometrically sound instruments.

Table 19

Correlation of ASCIP, Beck Depression Inventory, Coping Strategies Questionnaire, Social Support Questionnaire, Psychological well-being Questionnaire and Quality of Life Questionnaire (n=500)

	1	2	3	4	5	6	7	8	9	10	11	12	13	14	15	16	17	18	19	20	21	22	23	24
1	-	.21**	.11*	.07	-.16**	-.02	-.15**	-.06	.07	.01	-.12**	-.09*	-.06	-.43**	-.35**	-.44**	.35**	-.45**	-.43**	.06	-.11**	.06	-.09*	.09*
2		-	-.11**	.33**	-.49**	-.09*	.04	.10*	-.19**	-.32**	-.53**	-.54**	-.27**	.07	.02	-.03	.06	-.06	.02	.00	-.20**	-.19**	-.23**	.38**
3			-	-.07*	-.17**	.03	-.44**	-.38**	.08*	.01	.20**	.17**	.04	-.12**	.07	-.14**	-.09*	-.11**	-.09*	-.06	-.10*	-.13**	-.14**	-.03
4				-	-.21**	.08*	.14**	.06	.05	-.04	.04	-.06	.19**	.04	.07	-.05	-.01	-.01	-.05	.19**	.25**	.02	.23**	-.09*
5					-	.23**	.27**	.42**	.26**	.54**	.62**	.73**	.55**	-.13**	-.15**	-.01	.04	.14**	-.14**	.15**	.36**	.58**	.63**	-.28**
6						-	.43**	.32**	.40**	.25**	.43**	.28**	.33**	-.02	-.05	.07	.08*	-.02	-.02	.51**	.19**	.22**	.59**	-.36**
7							-	.53**	-.03	.02	.02	-.01	.26**	.16**	-.09*	.19**	.07	.27**	.07	.35**	.34**	.29**	.53**	-.03
8								-	.26**	.32**	.05	.04	.15**	-.06	-.09*	-.07	-.02	.05	-.12**	.24**	.14**	.40**	.56**	-.08*
9									-	.46**	.54**	.44**	.33**	-.30**	-.17**	-.22**	.21**	-.36**	-.28**	.17**	.13**	.32**	.42**	-.38**
10										-	.58**	.57**	.40**	-.31**	-.18**	-.25**	.13**	-.19**	-.30**	.18**	.33**	.39**	.50**	-.40**
11											-	.92**	.73**	-.17**	-.08*	-.03	.13**	-.08*	-.13**	.31**	.40**	.44**	.70**	-.60**
12												-	.77**	-.21**	-.09*	-.07	.14**	-.06	-.20**	.25**	.37**	.52**	.67**	-.51**
13													-	-.13**	-.12**	-.05	.20**	.00	-.21**	.52**	.60**	.59**	.83**	-.12**
14														-	.86**	.92**	-.72**	.87**	.92**	-.14**	.01	-.32**	-.10*	.04
15															-	.69**	-.89**	.71**	.72**	-.11**	-.07	-.28**	-.12**	-.09*
16																-	-.52**	.83**	.96**	-.11**	.01	-.23**	-.02	-.07
17																	-	-.72**	-.58**	.16**	.06	.25**	.15**	-.01
18																		-	.81**	-.12**	.16**	-.12**	.04	.07
19																			-	-.19**	-.07*	-.35**	-.17**	-.06
20																				-	.33**	.37**	.60**	-.11**
21																					-	.36**	.58**	-.09*
22																						-	.65**	-.14**
23																							-	-.38**
24																								-

Note. 1= Beck Depression Inventory, 2 = State Anger, 3 = Anger Control-in, 4 = Anger Control-Out, 5 = Active–Focused Coping Strategies, 6 = Distracting–Focused Coping Strategies, 7 = Avoidance Focused Coping Strategies, 8 = Religious–Focused Coping Strategies, 9 Informational Support, 10 = Tangible Support, 11 = Emotional Support, 12 = Esteem Support, 13 = Social Network Support, 14 = Environmental Mastery, 15 = Self-Acceptance,16 = Positive relations with others, 17 = Autonomy, 18 = Purpose in life, 19 = Personal Growth, 20 = Physical functioning, 21 = Psychological Functioning , 22 = Social relationships, 23 = Environment, 24 = Perception of quality of life and health.

Table 19 shows the bivariate correlation matrix of all the scales. It shows a distinct pattern of significant positive and negative relationship between different variables. It indicates a significant positive relationship between the depression and the state anger. Depression has significant negative relationship with the active – focused coping strategies, avoidance – focused coping strategies, emotional support, esteem support, environmental mastery, self-acceptance, positive relations with others, autonomy, purpose in life, personal growth, psychological functioning and environment. State anger is significantly negatively correlated with the anger control-in but positively correlated with control-out. Religious focused coping strategies are positively related with the tangiable support, social network support, informational support, physical functioning, psychological functioning, social relations and environment. Furthermore, the results in this table indicates that as the avoidance focused coping strategies increases the religious focused coping strategies also increases. Avoidance –focused coping strategies also has a significant negative relationship with the social network support, environmental mastery, self-acceptance, positive relations with others, purpose in life, physical function, psychological functioning, social relationships and environment.

Table 20

Correlation of ASCIP, Beck Depression Inventory, Coping Strategies Questionnaire, Social Support Questionnaire, Psychological well-being Questionnaire and Quality of Life Questionnaire of Diabetic and Cancer Patients (n=104, 196)

	1	2	3	4	5	6	7	8	9	10	11	12	13	14	15	16	17	18	19	20	21	22	23	24
1	-	.81**	.18*	.26**	-.87**	-.38**	-.30**	-.40**	-.25**	-.27**	-.73**	-.71**	-.46**	.14	.06	-.41**	.10	-.41**	-.14	-.18*	-.19*	-.52**	-.70**	.76**
2	.73**	-	-.21*	.40**	-.79**	-.26**	.07	.16	-.20*	-.28**	-.85**	-.84**	-.53**	.42**	-.03	-.19*	.24**	-.32**	.00	-.20*	-.21*	-.41**	-.49**	.72**
3	.46**	-.06	-	-.22*	-.03	.08	-.61**	-.47**	.12	.11	.39**	.38**	.20*	-.58**	.25**	-.48**	-.28**	-.26**	-.32**	-.06	-.04	-.10	-.07	-.11
4	.18**	.27**	-.05	-	-.48**	.04	.21*	.14	-.12	.07	-.16	-.26**	.07	.18*	.13	-.43**	-.03	-.13	-.32**	.20*	.15	-.11	.17*	-.03
5	-.84**	-.72**	-.44**	-.32**	-	.36**	.22*	.29**	.28**	.26**	.76**	.80**	.66**	-.08	-.09	.48**	.04	.45**	.05	.20*	.19*	.56**	.70**	-.46**
6	-.21**	-.17*	.06	.10	.20**	-	.43**	.28**	.27**	.21*	.42**	.32**	.39**	-.05	-.02	.02	-.08	.16	-.23*	.53**	.20*	.33**	.60**	-.28**
7	-.40**	.01	-.62**	.17**	.38**	.34**	-	.48**	-.11	.00	-.07	-.06	.14	.28**	-.40**	.19*	.33**	.33**	-.19*	.32**	.22*	.13	.44**	-.03
8	-.57**	.08	-.66**	.07	.43**	.19**	.50**	-	.29**	.12	.03	-.01	.10	.44**	.07	.36**	.03	.07	.14	.01	-.09	.38**	.50**	-.11
9	-.33**	-.32**	.14*	.25**	.18**	.28**	-.03	.25**	-	.18*	.36**	.32**	.29**	.31**	.52**	-.00	-.39**	-.13	-.12	.13	.01	.67**	.34**	-.19*
10	-.72**	-.69**	-.04	-.16*	.67**	.18**	-.03	.34**	.33**	-	.43**	.37**	.41**	-.02	.26**	-.15	-.22*	.01	-.20*	.10	.33**	.26**	.40**	-.26**
11	-.57**	-.82**	.26**	.14*	.57**	.28**	-.03	-.03	.50**	.71**	-	.95**	.80**	-.34**	.20*	-.02	-.28**	.27**	-.27**	.29**	.28**	.51**	.75**	-.69**
12	-.55**	-.80**	.17**	-.03	.68**	.15*	-.06	-.01	.38**	.76**	.92**	-	.81**	-.29**	.22*	-.03	-.28**	.31**	-.33**	.22*	.25**	.55**	.72**	-.64**
13	-.29**	-.39**	-.05	.35**	.51**	.19**	.23**	.08	.25**	.43**	.71**	.74**	-	-.00	.17*	-.07	-.06	.27**	-.52**	.40**	.41**	.57**	.84**	-.29**
14	.05	.35**	-.60**	-.01	.14*	-.16*	.22**	.37**	-.10	-.14*	-.42**	-.19**	.08	-	.27**	.25**	.03	.04	.03	.14	-.01	.39**	.10	.38**
15	.21**	.03	.30**	.11	-.22**	-.03	-.45**	-.08	.35**	.16*	.10	.20**	.11	.22**	-	-.40**	-.82**	-.43**	-.33**	-.08	-.15	.48**	.11	-.21*
16	-.50**	-.22**	-.54**	-.46**	.51**	-.00	.21**	.42**	-.08	.19**	-.12*	-.07	-.20**	.35**	-.35**	-	.38**	.43**	.66**	-.02	-.10	.17*	.08	.05
17	-.06	.14*	-.37**	.05	.16*	-.13*	.39**	.05	-.38**	-.19**	-.16*	-.19**	.06	.10	-.83**	.31**	-	.19*	.32**	.08	.20*	-.32**	-.06	.39**
18	-.43**	-.24**	-.34**	-.18**	.51**	.13*	.32**	.30**	-.06	.24**	.16*	.22**	.21**	.18**	-.48**	.56**	.36**	-	.09	.19*	.12	.15	.32**	-.13
19	-.23**	-.00	-.23**	-.49**	.03	-.24**	-.19**	.19**	-.21**	.03	-.360**	-.39**	-.66**	.02	-.31**	.65**	.21**	.20**	-	-.26**	-.25**	-.20*	-.35**	-.02
20	-.06	.02	-.12	.22**	.11	.37**	.20**	.22**	-.02	.16*	.16*	.17**	.40**	.22**	.31**	-.13*	-.23**	-.01	-.35**	-	.17*	.27**	.46**	-.12
21	-.33**	-.33**	-.24**	.50**	.39**	.11	.31**	.08	.21**	.23**	.56**	.49**	.75**	.02	-.17**	-.04	.34**	.23**	-.40**	.28**	-	.08	.36**	-.10
22	-.41**	-.29**	-.30**	.00	.48**	.03	.28**	.26**	.01	.28**	.30**	.34**	.40**	.15*	-.18**	.29**	.18**	.39**	-.05	.07	.36**	-	.65**	-.34**
23	-.62**	-.40**	-.33**	.38**	.65**	.40**	.50**	.52**	.36**	.58**	.68**	.65**	.83**	.10	-.02	.03	.10	.32**	-.44**	.45**	.70**	.44**	-	-.51**
24	.61**	.66**	-.07	-.15*	-.36**	-.15*	.08	-.14*	-.50**	-.66**	-.69**	-.60**	-.19**	.39**	-.15*	.04	.23**	.06	-.01	.00	-.29**	-.12	-.42**	-

Note. The values above the diagonal show correlation coefficient for diabetic patients and below the diagonal show correlation for the cancer patients.

1= Beck Depression Inventory, 2 = State Anger, 3 = Anger Control-in, 4 = Anger Control-Out, 5 = Active–Focused Coping Strategies, 6 = Distracting–Focused Coping Strategies, 7 = Avoidance Focused Coping Strategies, 8 = Religious–Focused Coping Strategies, 9 Informational Support, 10 = Tangible Support, 11 = Emotional Support, 12 = Esteem Support, 13 = Social Network Support, 14 = Environmental Mastery, 15 = Self-Acceptance,16 = Positive relations with others, 17 = Autonomy, 18 = Purpose in life, 19 = Personal Growth, 20 = Physical functioning, 21 = Psychological Functioning , 22 = Social relationships, 23 = Environment, 24 = Perception of quality of life and health.

Table 20 shows the bivariate correlation matrix of all the scales. The values above the diagonal show correlation coefficient for diabetic patients and below the diagonal show correlation for the cancer patients. It shows a distinct pattern of significant positive and negative relationship between different variables. Depression has significant relationship with state anger, anger control-in and anger control-out, whereas significant negative relationship with the active focused coping strategies, active distracting coping strategies, avoidance focused coping strategies, religious focused coping strategies, informational support, tangible support, emotional support, esteem support, social relations, positive relations with others, purpose in life, physical functioning, psychological functioning, social relationships and environment. State anger has significant positive relationship with anger control-out, environmental mastery and autonomy whereas it has negative relationship with the active focused coping strategies, active distracting coping strategies, informational support, tangible support, emotional support, esteem support, social network support, positive relations, purpose in life, physical functioning, psychological functioning, social relations and environment. Anger control-in has significant negative relationship with anger control out, avoidance focused coping strategies, religious focused coping strategies, environmental mastery, positive relations with others, autonomy, purpose in life, and personal growth. Whereas it has positive relationship with the emotional support, esteem support, and social network support among diabetic patients.

Depression has significant positive relationship with the state anger, anger control-in, anger control-out, and self-acceptance. Whereas it (depression) has negative relationship with the active focused coping strategies, active distracting coping strategies, avoidance focused coping strategies, religious focused coping strategies, informational support, tangible support, emotional support, esteem support, social network support, positive relations with others, purpose in life, personal growth, psychological functioning, physical functioning, social relations and environment. State anger has significant positive relationship with the anger control-out, environmental mastery and autonomy. Whereas it has negative relationship with active focused coping strategies, informational support, esteem support, social network support, positive relations with others, purpose in life, physical functioning, psychological functioning, social relations and environment. Anger control-in is having a positive relationship with the informational support, emotional support, esteem support, and self-acceptance whereas anger control-out is having a positive relationship with the avoidance focused coping strategies, informational support, emotional support, social network support, physical functioning, psychological functioning and environment among cancer patients.

Table 21

Correlation of ASCIP, Beck Depression Inventory, Coping Strategies Questionnaire, Social Support Questionnaire, Psychological well-being Questionnaire and Quality of Life Questionnaire of Cardiac Patients (n=200)

	1	2	3	4	5	6	7	8	9	10	11	12	13	14	15	16	17	18	19	20	21	22	23	24
1	-	.04	.01	.06	.10	.10	.11	.06	.05	.10	.04	.09	.05	-.09	-.04	.00	.06	.00	-.06	.09	.06	.14*	.12*	-.14*
2		-	-.11	.34**	-.07	.08	.11	.08	-.02	-.05	-.09	-.10	-.03	.06	.07	.06	-.02	.04	.09	.10	-.02	.02	.05	-.05
3			-	-.04	.03	-.03	-.02	-.04	.01	.01	.05	.06	.05	-.06	-.09	-.03	.05	-.03	-.04	-.01	.03	.01	.00	.04
4				-	.06	.09	.04	.01	.06	.07	.07	.05	.11	-.04	-.04	.04	.04	-.04	.05	.17**	.11	.12*	.13*	-.07
5					-	.19**	.18**	.49**	.36**	.88**	.58**	.74**	.55**	-.72**	-.39**	-.61**	-.04	.17**	-.74**	.17**	.60**	.73**	.58**	-.10
6						-	.65**	.51**	.84**	.55**	.59**	.40**	.44**	-.11	-.32**	.31**	.43**	-.41**	.13*	.66**	.32**	.38**	.76**	-.61**
7							-	.75**	.28**	.34**	.18**	.16*	.45**	-.42**	-.38**	-.19**	.21**	.05	-.39**	.77**	.61**	.66**	.77**	-.18**
8								-	.24**	.58**	.13*	.11	.25**	-.27**	-.08	-.49**	-.30**	.44**	-.54**	.39**	.56**	.55**	.64**	-.00
9									-	.67**	.85**	.69**	.59**	-.20**	-.49**	.37**	.58**	-.61**	.16*	.45**	.25**	.33**	.67**	-.53**
10										-	.80**	.80**	.58**	-.56**	-.35**	-.36**	.14*	-.12*	-.52**	.35**	.54**	.71**	.75**	-.41**
11											-	.90**	.73**	-.52**	-.58**	.04	.59**	-.63**	-.16*	.47**	.44**	.55**	.68**	-.48**
12												-	.78**	-.72**	-.70**	-.08	.61**	-.49**	-.39**	.35**	.44**	.68**	.66**	-.36**
13													-	-.78**	-.91**	-.20	.62**	-.38**	-.38**	.73**	.78**	.81**	.83**	.02
14														-	.78**	.53**	-.36**	.06	.79**	-.49**	-.77**	-.87**	-.65**	-.03
15															-	-.00	-.69**	.37**	.33**	-.58**	-.66**	-.66**	-.66**	-.11
16																-	.56**	-.62**	.88**	-.02	-.55**	-.48**	-.16**	-.30**
17																	-	-.85**	.20**	.48**	.10	.30**	.43**	-.38**
18																		-	-.45**	-.32**	.14*	-.01	-.21**	.54**
19																			-	-.17**	-.66**	-.73**	-.42**	-.21**
20																				-	.75**	.71**	.85**	-.22**
21																					-	.86**	.80**	.19**
22																						-	.88**	-.09
23																							-	-.28**
24																								-

Note. 1= Beck Depression Inventory, 2 = State Anger, 3 = Anger Control-in, 4 = Anger Control-Out, 5 = Active–Focused Coping Strategies, 6 = Distracting–Focused Coping Strategies, 7 = Avoidance Focused Coping Strategies, 8 = Religious–Focused Coping Strategies, 9 Informational Support, 10 = Tangible Support, 11 = Emotional Support, 12 = Esteem Support, 13 = Social Network Support, 14 = Environmental Mastery, 15 = Self-Acceptance,16 = Positive relations with others, 17 = Autonomy, 18 = Purpose in life, 19 = Personal Growth, 20 = Physical functioning, 21 = Psychological Functioning , 22 = Social relationships, 23 = Environment, 24 = Perception of quality of life and health.

Table 21 shows the bivariate correlation matrix of all the scales. It shows a distinct pattern of significant positive and negative relationship between different variables. Depression has significant positive relationship between the social relations and environment, whereas it has significant negative with the perception of quality of life and health. State anger has significant positive relationship with anger control-in.

Prevalence of Psychological Issues

Table 22

Comparison on level of depression, state anger-in and state anger-out among diabetic, cancer and cardiac patients (N = 500).

	Diabetics (N = 104)		Cancer (N = 196)		Cardiac (N = 200)		F	p	η^2	i-j	Mean (i-j)	SE	95% CI	
	M	SD	M	SD	M	SD							LL	UL
Depression	11.52	5.97	9.72	5.37	22.89	18.35	62.18	.000	.20	D>Can	1.80	1.50	-1.73	5.33
										D<Car	-11.37*	1.50	-14.89	-7.84
										Can<D	-1.80	1.50	-5.33	1.73
										Can<Car	-13.17*	1.25	-16.09	-1.24
										Car>D	11.37*	1.50	7.84	14.89
										Car>Can	13.17*	1.25	10.24	16.09
State anger	13.70	5.72	12.51	4.51	12.92	4.99	1.95	.14						
Anger control-in	20.92	6.45	20.17	7.06	20.79	6.83	.58	.56						
Anger control-out	7.85	2.64	7.46	2.65	7.36	2.80	1.14	.32						

Results in the Table 22 indicates that ANOVA was computed for the exploration of mean differences on depression, state anger, anger control-in and anger control-out among diabetic, cancer and cardiac patients. Results indicate that there is a significant difference among diabetic, cardiac and cancer patients on depression. It is high among cardiac patients as compared to diabetic and cancer patients. Post-hoc analysis indicates that there is a significant difference of level of depression among diabetic and cardiac patients as it is high among cardiac as compared to diabetics, results also indicated that there is a significant difference among cardiac and cancer patients on level of depression as it is high among cardiac patients as compared to cancer patients.

Table 23

Chi-Square of level of depression among diabetic, cancer and cardiac patients (N = 500)

Level of Depression	Diabetic patients ($N = 104$)	Cancer patients ($N = 196$)	Cardiac patients ($N = 200$)	X^2	p
Normal ups and downs	52 (50%)	128 (65.3%)	72 (36%)		
Mild	38 (36.5%)	52 (26.5%)	28 (14%)		
Borderline	0 (0%)	1 (.5%)	4 (47%)		
Moderate	14 (13.5%)	15 (7.7%)	47 (23.5%)		
Severe	0 (0%)	0 (0%)	17 (8.5 %)	126.40	.00
Extreme	0 (0%)	0 (0%)	32 (16.0%)		

The results in the Table 23 indicate that the level of depression varies among diabetic, cancer and cardiac patients this difference is statistically significant.

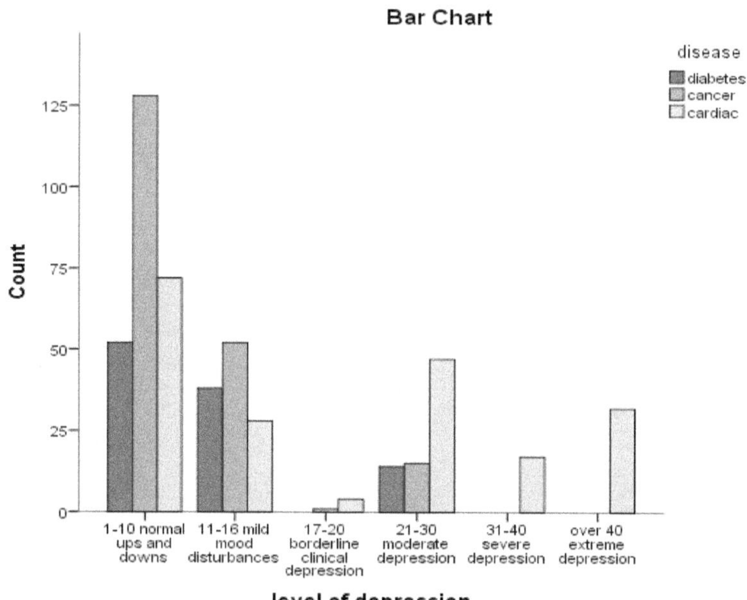

Figure 2. Level of depression among diabetic, cancer and cardiac patients

Table 24

Chi-Square of level of Depression among Male and Female Diabetic Patients (N =104)

Level of depression	Males (N =54)	Female (N =50)	X^2	p
normal ups and downs	31 (57.41%)	21 (42%)		
mild	14 (25.93%)	24 (48%)	5.55	.06
moderate	9 (16.67%)	5 (10%)		

The results in the Table 24 indicate that the level of depression varies among male and female diabetes patients but that is not statistically significant.

Table 25

Chi-Square of level of Depression among Male and Female Cancer Patients (N =196)

Level of depression	Males (N =4)	Female (N = 192)	X^2	p
normal ups and downs	4 (100%)	124 (64.58%)		
mild	0 (0%)	52 (27.08%)		
borderline	0 (0%)	1(0.52%)	2.17	.54
moderate	0 (0%)	15 (7.81%)		

The results in the Table 25 indicate that the level of depression varies among patients but that is not statistically significant among male and female cancer patients.

Table 26

Chi-Square of Level of Depression among Male and Female Cardiac Patients (N =200)

Level of depression	Males (N =73)	Female (N = 127)	X^2	p
Normal ups and downs	32 (43.84%)	40 (31.50%)		
Mild	9 (12.33%)	19 (14.96%)		
Borderline	2 (2.74%)	2 (1.57%)	5.70	.33
Moderate	16 (21.92%)	31 (24.41%)		
Severe	7 (9.59%)	10 (7.87%)		
Extreme	7 (9.59%)	25 (19.69%)		

The results in the Table 26 indicated that the level of depression is not statistically significantly different among different male and female cardiac patients.

Table 27

Chi-Square of Level of State Anger among Diabetic, Cancer and Cardiac Patients (N = 500)

Level of state anger	Diabetic patients ($N = 104$)	Cancer patients ($N = 196$)	Cardiac patients ($N = 200$)	X^2	p
Moderate	71 (68.3%)	162 (82.7)	154 (77%)	8.07	.02
Severe	33 (31.7%)	34 (17.3)	46 (33%)		

The results in the Table 27 indicate that the level of state anger varies among diabetic, cancer and cardiac patients this difference is statistically significant.

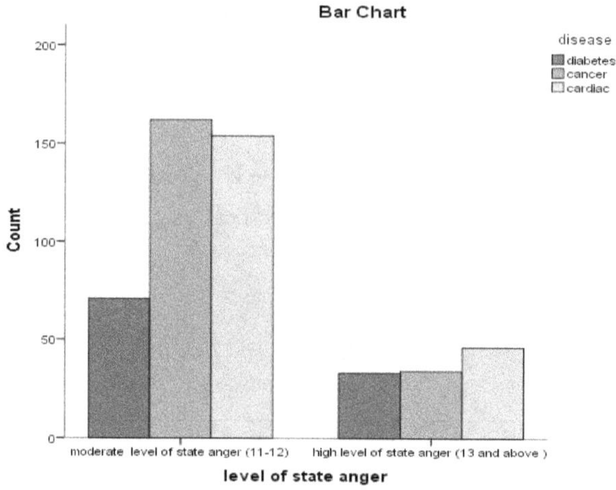

Figure 3. Level of State anger among diabetic, cancer and cardiac patients

Table 28

Chi-Square of Level of State Anger among Male and Female Diabetic Patients (N = 104)

Level of state anger	Male ($N = 54$)	Female ($N = 50$)	X^2	p
Moderate	40 (74.07%)	31 (62%)		
Severe	14 (25.93%)	19 (38%)	1.75	.19

The results in the Table 28 indicate that the level of state anger varies among diabetic male and female patients but that is not statistically significant.

Table 29

Chi-Square of Level of State Anger among Male and Female Cancer Patients (N = 196)

Level of state anger	Male ($N = 4$)	Female ($N = 192$)	X^2	p
Moderate	4(100%)	158 (82.29%)		
Severe	0 (0%)	34 (17.71%)	.86	.36

The results in the Table 29 indicate that the level of state anger varies among cancer male and female patients but that is not statistically significant.

Table 30

Chi-Square of Level of State Anger among Male and Female Cardiac Patients (N = 200)

Level of state anger	Male ($N = 73$)	Female ($N = 127$)	X^2	p
Moderate	54 (73.97%)	100(78.74%)		
Severe	19(26.03%)	27(21.26)	.6	.44

The results in the Table 30 indicate that the level of state anger varies among cardiac male and female patients but that is not statistically significant.

Table 31

Chi-Square of Level of Anger Control-in among Diabetic, Cancer and Cardiac Patients (N = 500)

Level of control-in	Diabetic patients ($N = 104$)	Cancer patients ($N = 196$)	Cardiac Patients ($N=200$)	X^2	p
Low	15 (14.4%)	46 (23.5%)	39 (19.5%)		
Moderate	67 (64.4%)	117 (59.7%)	115 (57.5%)	5.29	.26
Severe	22 (21.2%)	33 (16.8%)	46 (23%)		

Results in the above Table 31 indicate the difference between the level of anger control-in among diabetic, cancer and cardiac patients but its not statistically significant.

Table 32

Chi-Square of Level of Anger Control-in among Male and Female Diabetic Patients (N = 104)

Level of control-in	Male ($N = 54$)	Female ($N = 50$)	X^2	p
Low	11 (20.37%)	4 (8%)		
Moderate	34 (62.96%)	33 (66%)	3.86	.15
Severe	9 (16.67%)	13 (26%)		

Results in the above Table 32 indicate the difference between the level of anger control-in among male and female diabetic patients but its not statistically significant.

Table 33

Chi-Square of Level of Anger Control-in among Male and Female Cancer Patients (N = 196)

Level of control-in	Male (N = 4)	Female (N = 192)	X^2	p
Low	4 (100%)	42 (28.88%)		
Moderate	0 (0%)	117 (60.94%)	13.32	.001
Severe	0 (0%)	33 (17.19%)		

Results in the above Table 33 indicate the difference between the level of anger control-in among male and female cancer patients and is statistically significantly high among female patients.

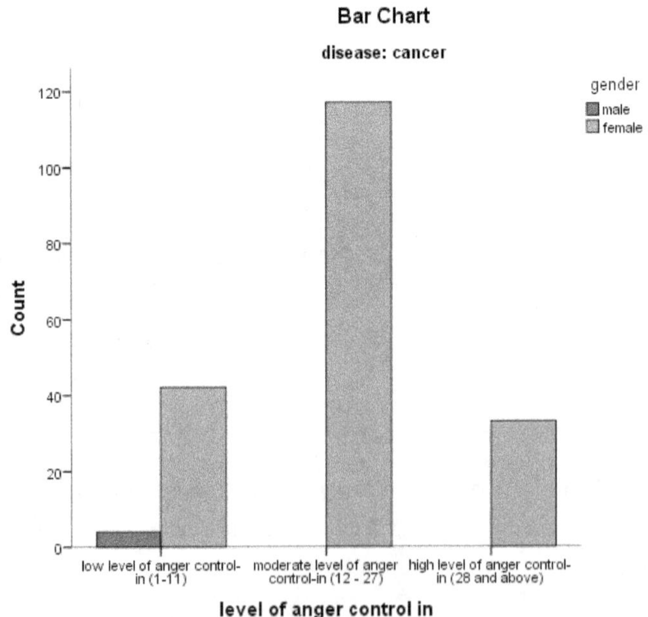

Figure 4. Level of anger control-in among male and female cancer patients

Table 34

Chi-Square of Level of Anger Control-in among Male and Female Cardiac Patients (N = 200)

Level of control-in	Male (N = 73)	Female (N = 127)	X^2	p
Low	19 (26.03%)	20 (15.75%)		
Moderate	37 (50.68%)	78 (61.42%)	3.45	.18
Severe	17 (23.29%)	29 (22.83%)		

Results in the above Table 34 indicate the difference between the level of anger control-in among male and female cardiac patients but its not statistically significant.

Table 35

Chi-Square of Level of Anger Control-out among Diabetic, Cancer and Cardiac Patients (N = 500)

Level of control-out	Diabetic patients (N = 104)	Cancer patients (N = 196)	Cardiac patients (N = 200)	X^2	p
Low	20 (19.2%)	52 (26.5%)	64 (32.0%)		
Moderate	65 (62.5%)	19 (55.6%)	99 (49.5%)	6.36	.17
Severe	19 (18.3%)	35 (17.9%)	37(18.5%)		

Results in the above Table 35 indicate the difference between the level of anger control-out among diabetic, cancer and cardiac patients but its not statistically significant.

Table 36

Chi-Square of Level of Anger Control-out among Male and Female Diabetic Patients
(N = 104)

Level of control-out	Male ($N = 54$)	Female ($N = 50$)	X^2	p
Low	12 (22.22%)	8 (16%)		
Moderate	31 (54.41%)	34 (68%)	1.26	.53
Severe	11 (20.37%)	8 (16%)		

Results in the above Table 36 indicate the difference between the level of anger control-out among male and female diabetic patients but its not statistically significant.

Table 37

Chi-Square of Level of Anger Control-out among Male and Female Cancer Patients
(N = 196)

Level of control-out	Male ($N = 4$)	Female ($N = 192$)	X^2	p
Low	4 (100%)	48 (25%)		
Moderate	0 (0%)	109 (56.77%)	11.31	.00
Severe	0 (0%)	35 (18.23%)		

Results in the above Table 37 indicates the difference between the level of anger control-out among male and female cancer patients and is significantly high among female patients.

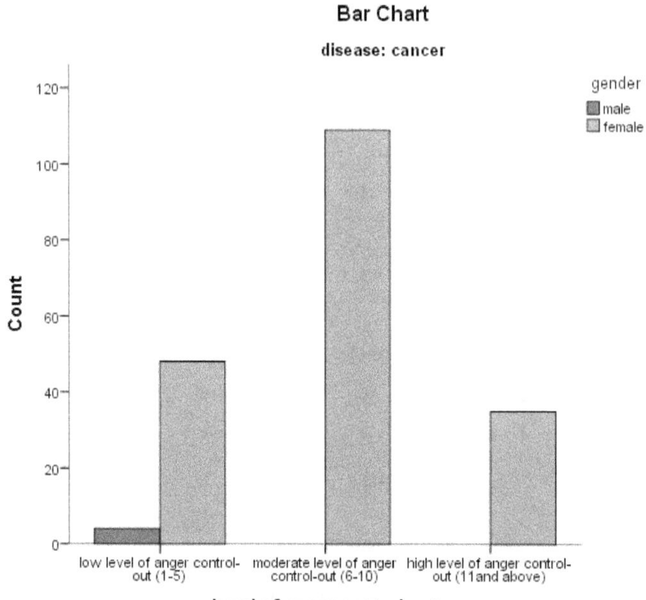

Figure 5. Level of anger control-out among male and female cancer patients

Table 38

Chi-Square of Level of Anger Control-Out among Male and Female Cardiac Patients
(N = 200)

Level of control-out	Male ($N = 73$)	Female ($N = 127$)	X^2	p
Low	25 (36.25%)	39 (30.71%)		
Moderate	38 (52.05%)	61 (48.03%)	1.77	.41
Severe	10 (13.70%)	27 (21.26%)		

Results in the above Table 38 indicate the difference between the level of anger control-out among male and female cardiac patients but its not statistically significant

Predictive role of Depression and Anger

Table 39

Multiple Regression Analysis Showing the Main Effects of Depression, State Anger, Anger Control-in and Anger Control-Out in the Prediction of Environmental Mastery among Chronically Ill Patients (N= 500)

Model	B	SE	β	t	p	95% CI LL	UL	Tolerance	VIF
Constant	34.98	2.722		12.85	.000	29.63	40.32		
Depression	-.47	.04	-.46	11.26	.000	-.56	-.39	.94	1.06
State anger	.43	.12	.15	3.52	.000	.19	.67	.85	1.18
Anger Control-in	-.12	.08	-.06	1.44	.15	-.28	.04	.97	1.03
Anger Control-out	.09	.00	.02	.42	.38	-.34	.52	.89	1.12

Table 39 is exhibiting the results of multiple regression analysis. In which the depression, state anger, anger control-in and anger control-out were entered as predictor variables, whereas the environmental mastery was entered as an outcome variable. The resultant model is explaining the 21.9% (R^2 = .219, p = .000) variance with significant beta values (β = -.46, p = .000) for depression and (β =.15, p = .000) for state anger.

Table 40

Multiple Regression Analysis Showing the Main Effects of Depression, State Anger, Anger Control-in and Anger Control-Out in the Prediction of Autonomy among Chronically Ill Patients (N= 500)

Model	B	SE	β	t	p	95%CI		Tolerance	VIF
						LL	UL		
Constant	35.69	2.24		15.92	.000	31.29	40.10		
Depression	.29	.03	.36	8.50	.00	.23	.36	.94	1.06
State anger	-.34	.10	-.02	.34	.73	-.23	.16	.85	1.18
Anger Control-in	-.22	.07	-.14	3.20	.001	-.36	-.09	.97	1.03
Anger Control-out	-.16	.18	-.04	.90	.37	-.52	.19	.89	1.12

Table 40 is exhibiting the results of multiple regression analysis. In which the depression, state anger, anger control-in and anger control-out were entered as predictor variables, whereas the autonomy was entered as an outcome variable. The resultant model is explaining the 13.8% ($R^2 = .138$, $p = .000$) variance with significant beta values ($\beta = .37$, $p = .000$) for depression and ($\beta = -.14$, $p = .000$) for anger control-in.

Table 41

Multiple Regression Analysis Showing the Main Effects of Depression, State Anger, Anger Control-in and Anger Control-Out in the Prediction of Personal Growth among Chronically Ill Patients (N= 500)

Model	B	SE	β	t	p	95%CI		Tolerance	VIF
						LL	UL		
Constant	35.58	2.09		17.02	.000	31.47	39.69		
Depression	-.36	.03	-.46	11.06	.000	-.42	-.29	.94	1.06
State anger	.28	.09	.13	2.96	.003	.09	.46	.85	1.18
Anger Control-in	-.06	.06	-.04	.91	.36	-.19	.07	.97	1.03
Anger Control-out	-.26	.17	-.07	1.56	.12	.60	.07	.89	1.12

Table 41 is exhibiting the results of multiple regression analysis. In which the depression, state anger, anger control-in and anger control-out were entered as a predictor variable, whereas the personal growth was entered as an outcome variable. The resultant model is explaining the 20.8% (R^2 = .208, p = .000) variance with significant beta values (β = -.46, p = .000) for depression and (β =.13, p = .003) for state anger.

Table 42

Multiple Regression Analysis Showing the Main Effects of Depression, State Anger, Anger Control-in and Anger Control-Out in the Prediction of Positive Relations with others among Chronically Ill Patients (N= 500)

Model	B	SE	β	t	p	95%CI		Tolerance	VIF
						LL	UL		
Constant	41.77	2.14		19.52	.000	37.56	45.97		
Depression	-.36	.03	-.45	10.87	.000	-.42	-.29	.94	1.06
State anger	.14	.10	.07	1.49	.14	-.05	.33	.84	1.18
Anger Control-in	-.15	.07	-.09	2.30	.02	-.28	-.02	.97	1.03
Anger Control-out	-.20	.17	-.05	1.15	.25	-.54	.14	.89	1.12

Table 42 is exhibiting the results of multiple regression analysis. In which the depression, state anger, anger control-in and anger control-out were entered as predictor variables, whereas the positive relations with others was entered as an outcome variable. The resultant model is explaining the 21.3% ($R^2 = .213$, $p = .000$) variance with significant beta values ($\beta = .03$, $p = .000$) for depression and ($\beta =-.09$, $p = .02$) for anger control-in.

Table 43

Multiple Regression Analysis Showing the Main Effects of Depression, State Anger, Anger Control-in and Anger Control-Out in the Prediction of Purpose in Life among Chronically Ill Patients (N= 500)

Model	B	SE	β	t	p	95%CI		Tolerance	VIF
						LL	UL		
Constant	37.24	2.06		18.06	.000	33.19	41.29		
Depression	-.35	.03	-.45	10.85	.000	-.41	-.28	.94	1.06
State anger	.05	.09	.02	.52	.60	-.13	.23	.84	1.18
Anger Control-in	-.09	.06	-.06	1.38	.17	-.21	.04	.97	1.03
Anger Control-out	.04	.17	.01	.23	.82	-.29	.37	.89	1.12

Table 43 is exhibiting the results of multiple regression analysis. In which the depression, state anger, anger control-in and anger control-out were entered as predictor variables, whereas the purpose in life was entered as an outcome variable. The resultant model is explaining the 20.5% (R^2 = .205, p = .000) variance with significant beta values (β = -.45, p = .000) for depression.

Table 44

Multiple Regression Analysis Showing the Main Effects of Depression, State Anger, Anger Control-in and Anger Control-Out in the Prediction of Self-Acceptance among Chronically Ill Patients (N= 500)

Model	B	SE	β	t	p	95%CI LL	95%CI UL	Tolerance	VIF
Constant	28.97	2.31		12.55	.000	24.43	33.50		
Depression	-.32	.04	-.39	9.03	.00	-.39	-.25	.94	1.06
State anger	.20	.10	.09	1.92	.06	-.004	.41	.85	1.18
Anger Control-in	.21	.07	.13	2.97	.003	.07	.35	.97	1.03
Anger Control-out	.34	.19	.08	1.80	.07	-.03	.70	.89	1.12

Table 44 is exhibiting the results of multiple regression analysis. In which the depression, state anger, anger control-in and anger control-out were entered as predictor variables, whereas the self-acceptance was entered as an outcome variable. The resultant model is explaining the 15.1% (R^2 = .151, p = .000) variance with significant beta values (β = -.39, p = .000) for depression and (β =.13, p = .003) for anger control-in.

Table 45

Multiple Regression Analysis Showing the Main Effects of Depression, State Anger, Anger Control-in and Anger Control-Out in the Prediction of Physical Functioning among Chronically Ill Patients (N= 500)

Model	B	SE	β	t	p	95%CI		Tolerance	VIF
						LL	UL		
Constant	70.56	5.62		12.55	.000	59.51	81.61		
Depression	.14	.09	.07	1.59	.11	-.03	.31	.94	1.06
State anger	-.49	.25	-.09	1.92	.06	-.99	.01	.84	1.18
Anger Control-in	-.24	.17	-.06	1.37	.17	-.58	.10	.97	1.03
Anger Control-out	2.09	.46	.21	4.60	.000	1.20	2.99	.89	1.12

Table 45 is exhibiting the results of multiple regression analysis. In which the depression, state anger, anger control-in and anger control-out were entered as predictor variables, whereas the physical functioning was entered as an outcome variable. The resultant model is explaining the 4.9% (R^2 = .049, p = .000) variance with significant beta values (β = -.21, p = .000) for anger control-out.

Table 46

Multiple Regression Analysis Showing the Main Effects of Depression, State Anger, Anger Control-in and Anger Control-Out in the Prediction of Psychological Functioning among Chronically Ill Patients (N= 500)

Model	B	SE	β	t	p	95%CI		Tolerance	VIF
						LL	UL		
Constant	69.00	2.94		23.44	.000	63.22	74.78		
Depression	-.06	.05	-.053	1.26	.21	-.15	.03	.94	1.06
State anger	-.93	.13	-.31	7.04	.000	-1.19	-.67	.85	1.18
Anger Control-in	-.23	.09	-.10	2.50	.01	-.40	-.05	.97	1.03
Anger Control-out	1.91	.24	.35	8.04	.000	1.45	2.38	.89	1.12

Table 46 is exhibiting the results of multiple regression analysis. In which the depression, state anger, anger control-in and anger control-out were entered as predictor variables, whereas the psychological functioning was entered as an outcome variable. The resultant model is explaining the 16.6% ($R^2 = .166$, $p = .000$) variance with significant beta values ($\beta = -.31$, $p = .000$) for state anger, ($\beta = -.10$, $p = .01$) for anger control-in and ($\beta = .35$, $p = .000$) for anger control-out.

Table 47

Multiple Regression Analysis Showing the Main Effects of Depression, State Anger, Anger Control-in and Anger Control-Out in the Prediction of Social Relationships among Chronically Ill Patients (N= 500)

Model	B	SE	β	t	p	95%CI		Tolerance	VIF
						LL	UL		
Constant	52.68	3.12		16.87	.000	46.55	58.82		
Depression	.14	.05	.12	2.80	.01	.04	.23	.94	1.06
State anger	-.77	.14	-.26	5.45	.000	-1.04	-.49	.85	1.18
Anger Control-in	-.35	.10	-.16	3.67	.000	-.54	-.16	.97	1.03
Anger Control-out	.46	.25	.08	1.82	.07	-.04	.96	.89	1.12

Table 47 is exhibiting the results of multiple regression analysis. In which the depression, state anger, anger control-in and anger control-out were entered as predictor variables, whereas the social relationships was entered as an outcome variable. The resultant model is explaining the 7.7% (R^2 = .077, p = .000) variance with significant beta values (β = .12, p = .01) for depression, (β = -.26, p = .000) for state anger and (β = -.16, p = .000) for anger control-in.

Table 48

Multiple Regression Analysis Showing the Main Effects of Depression, State Anger, Anger Control-in and Anger Control-Out in the Prediction of Environment among Chronically Ill Patients (N= 500)

Model	B	SE	β	t	p	95%CI		Tolerance	VIF
						LL	UL		
Constant	128.44	5.57		23.08	.000	117.5	139.3		
Depression	-.04	.09	-.02	.47	.64	-.21	.13	.94	1.06
State anger	-2.01	.25	-.36	8.03	.000	-2.51	-1.52	.85	1.18
Anger Control-in	-.63	.17	-.15	3.71	.000	-.97	-.30	.97	1.03
Anger Control-out	3.45	.45	.33	7.76	.000	2.61	4.39	.89	1.12

Table 48 is exhibiting the results of multiple regression analysis. In which the depression, state anger, anger control-in and anger control-out were entered as predictor variables, whereas the environment was entered as an outcome variable. The resultant model is explaining the 18.2% ($R^2 = .182$, $p = .000$) variance with significant beta values ($\beta = -.36$, $p = .000$) for state anger, ($\beta = -.15$, $p = .000$) for anger control-in and ($\beta = .33$, $p = .000$) for anger control-out.

Moderating Role of Social Support and Coping Strategies

Table 49

Moderating Effect of active focused coping strategies on Relationship of Depression with Environmental Mastery, Self-Acceptance, Positive Relations, Purpose In Life, Autonomy and Personal Growth (n = 500)

| | Environmental | | | | | | | | | | | |
| | Mastery | | Self-acceptance | | Positive relation | | Purpose in life | | Personal growth | | Autonomy | |
Variables	ΔR^2	β	ΔR^2	β	ΔR^2	β	ΔR^2	β	ΔR^2	β	ΔR^2	β
Step 1												
Depression		-.39**		-.36**		-.38**		-.39**		-.41**		.37**
Active focused coping		-.15**		-.20**		-.03**		.11*		-.17**		.10*
Step 2	.07		.01		.08		.03**		.05		.00	
Depression * Active focused coping		-.30**		-.10**		-.32**		-.20**		-.26**		-.02
R^2	.27		.17		.28		.23		.26		.12	

** $p < .01$, * $p < .05$.

Table 49 illustrates moderation analysis for active coping strategies in the relationship of depression with psychological well-being (environmental mastery, self-acceptance, positive relations, purpose in life and personal growth). Active focused coping strategies are acting as a moderator for the relationship of depression with environmental mastery, autonomy, positive relations, purpose in life, self-acceptance, and personal growth. Moderation analysis for active coping strategies in the relationship between depression and autonomy doesn't occur. These added additional 7% variance is explained by the relationship (environmental mastery and depression) which is moderated by active focused coping strategies. It also added additional 1% variance is explained by the relationship (self-acceptance and depression) which is moderated by active focused coping strategies. It also added additional 8% variance is explained by the relationship (positive relations with others and depression) which is moderated by active focused coping strategies. It also added additional 3% variance is explained by the relationship (purpose in life and depression) which is moderated by active focused coping strategies. Furthermore, it also added additional 5% variance is explained by the relationship (personal growth and depression) which is moderated by active focused coping strategies. The moderating effect is further explained through mod graphs.

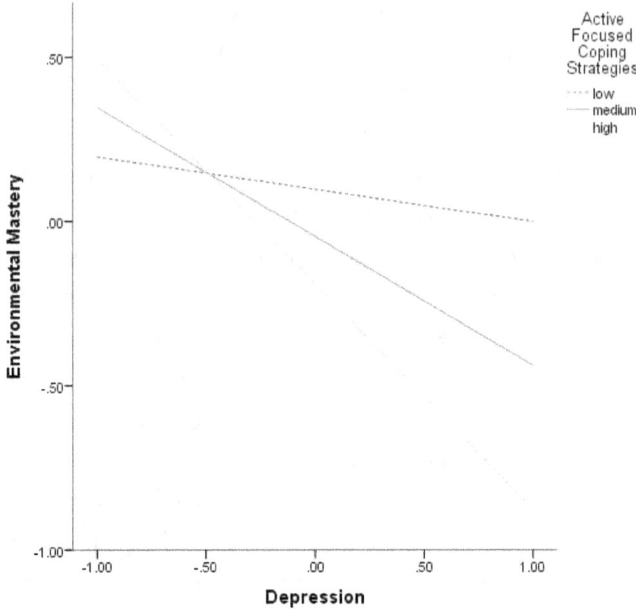

Figure 6. Active coping strategies as a moderator between environmental mastery and depression

Active focused coping strategies, moderated the relationship of depression with environmental mastery is moderated by the. When the active focused coping strategies are increasingly used by the patients, the association between depression and environmental mastery is negative, which means that in case if the patients are using the active focused coping strategies the depression increases and environmental mastery decreases.

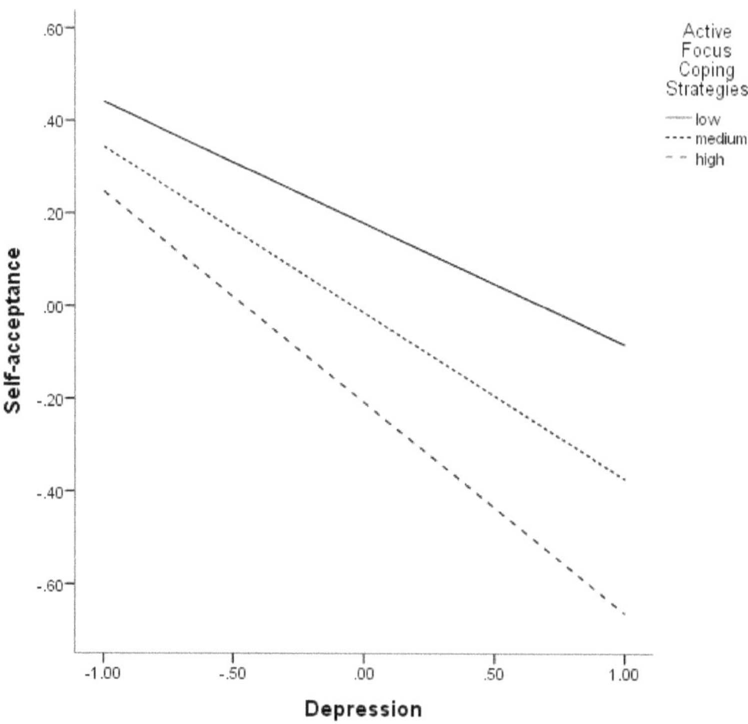

Figure 7. Active coping strategies as a moderator between Self-acceptance and depression

The correlation of depression with self-acceptance is moderated by the active focused coping strategies. When the active focused coping strategies are increasingly used by the patients, the relationship between depression and self-acceptance is negative, which means that in case if the patients are using the active focused coping strategies the depression increases and self-acceptance decreases.

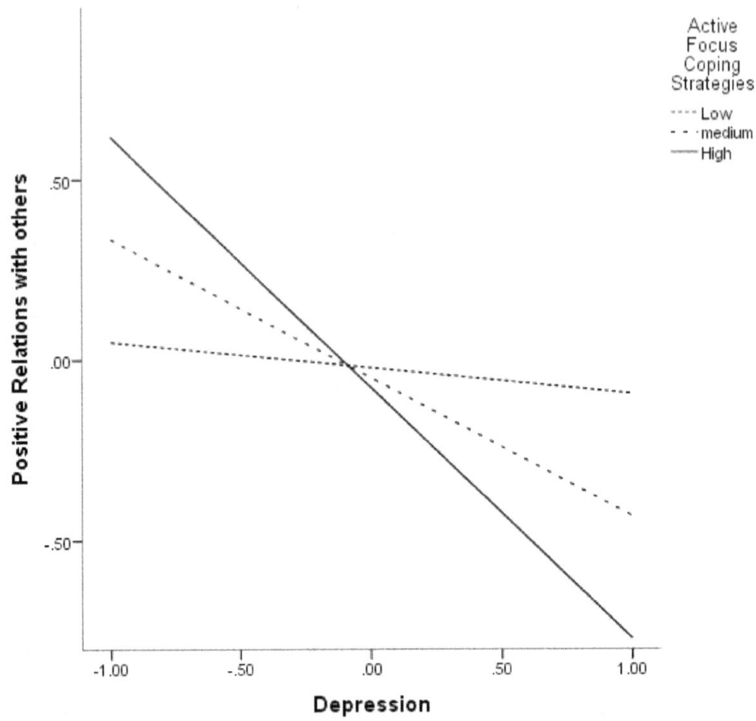

Figure 8. Active coping strategies as a moderator between the relationships of depression with positive relations with others

The correlation of depression and positive relations with others is moderated by the active focused coping strategies. When the active focused coping strategies are increasingly used by the patients, negative relationship of depression with positive relations with others, which means that in case if the patients are using the active focused coping strategies the depression increases and positive relations with others decreases.

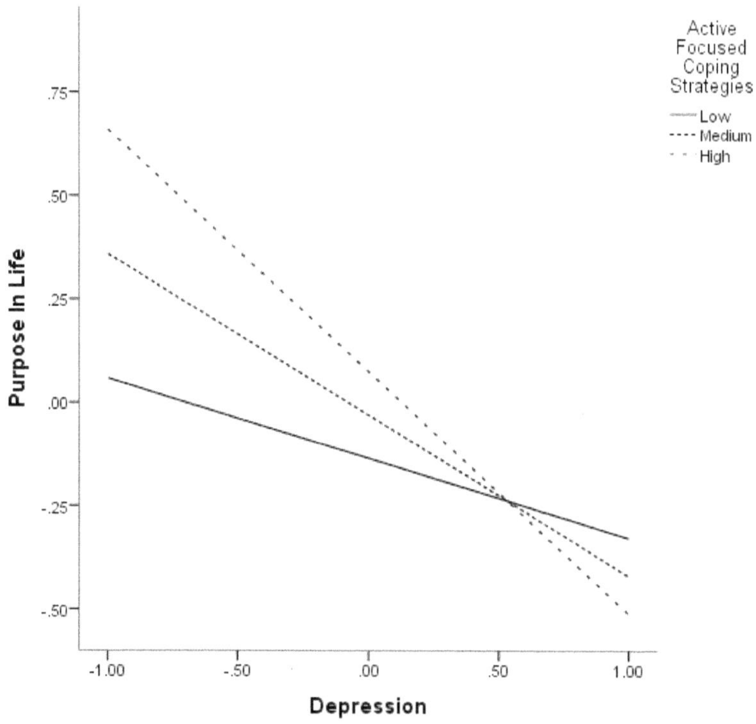

Figure 9. Active coping strategies as a moderator between purpose in life and depression

The correlation of depression with purpose in life is moderated by the active focused coping strategies. When the active focused coping strategies are increasingly used by the patients, the association of depression with purpose in life is negative, which means that in case if the patients are using the active focused coping strategies the depression increases and purpose in life decreases.

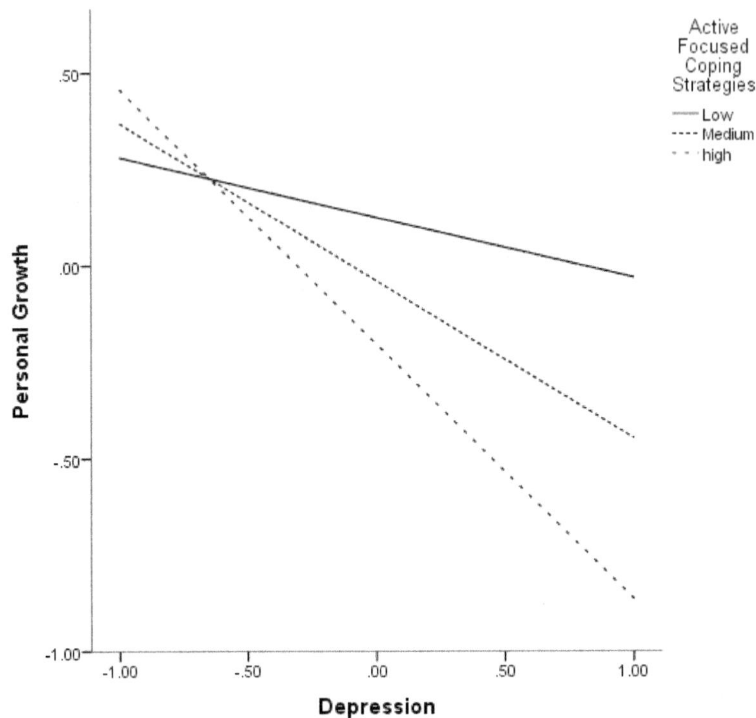

Figure 10. Active coping strategies as a moderator between personal growth and depression

The correlation of depression with personal growth is moderated by the active focused coping strategies. When the active focused coping strategies are increasingly used by the patients, the association of depression with personal growth is negative, which means that in case if the patients are using the active focused coping strategies the depression increases and personal growth decreases.

125

Table 50

Moderating Effect of active distracting coping strategies on Relationship of Depression with Environmental Mastery, Autonomy, Positive Relations, Purpose In Life, Self-Acceptance and Personal Growth (n = 500)

Variables	Environmental Mastery		Self-acceptance		Positive relation		Purpose in life		Personal growth		Autonomy	
	ΔR^2	β	ΔR^2	β	ΔR^2	β	ΔR^2	β	ΔR^2	β	ΔR^2	β
Step 1												
Depression		-.43**		-.33**		-.45		-.43**		-.45**		.31**
Active distracting coping		-.22		-.05		.05		-.02		-.02		.07
Step 2	.00		.01		.00		.01		.00		.04	
Depression * Active distracting coping		-.04		-.09**		.03		-.06**		.03		.15**
R^2	.19		.14		.20		.21		.19		.17	

** $p < .01$, * $p < .05$.

Table 50 illustrates moderation analysis for active-distracting coping strategies in the relationship between depression and Psychological well-being (environmental mastery, automny, self-acceptance, purpose in life, positive relations and personal growth). Active distracting coping strategies are acting as a moderator for the relationship of depression with self-acceptance, purpose in life, and autonomy. Moderation analysis for active coping strategies in the relationship between depression and environmental mastery, positive relations and personal growth doesn't occur. These added additional 1% variance is explained by the relationship (purpose in life and depression) which is moderated by active distracting coping strategies. It also added additional 4% variance is explained by the relationship (autonomy and depression) which is moderated by active distracting coping strategies. The moderating effect is further explained through mod graphs.

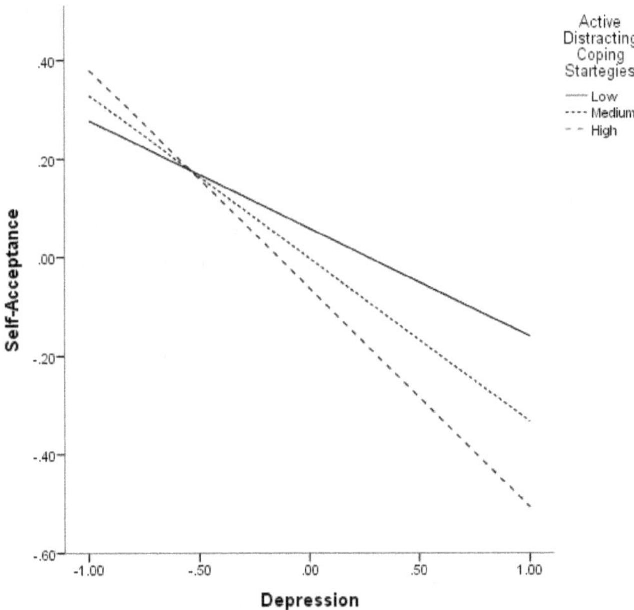

Figure 11. Active Distracting coping strategies as a moderator between self-acceptance and depression

The association between the depression and self-acceptance is moderated by the active distracting coping strategies. When the active distracting coping strategies are increasingly used by the patients, the association of depression with self-acceptance is negative, which means that in case if the patients are using the active distracting coping strategies the depression increases and self-acceptance decreases.

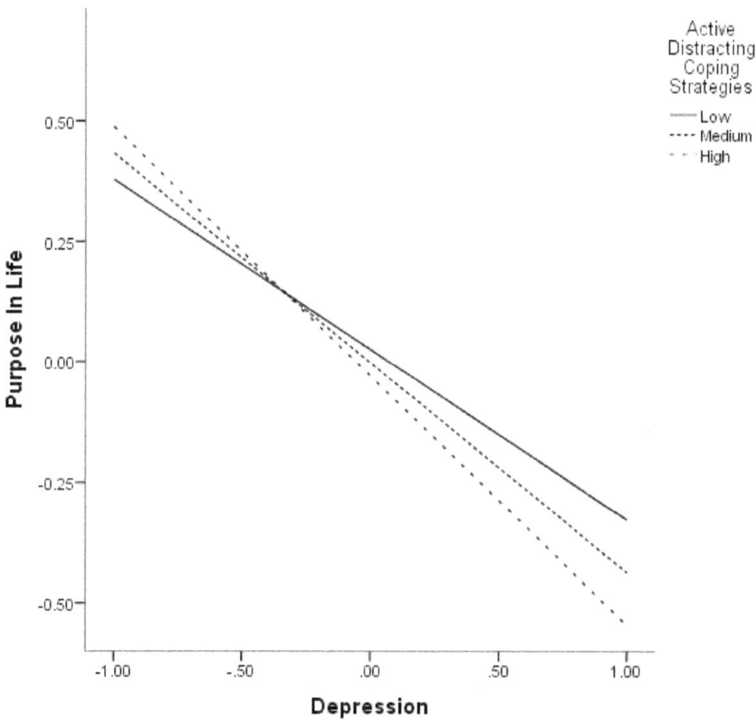

Figure 12. Active Distracting coping strategies as a moderator between purpose in life and depression

The relationship between the depression and purpose in life is moderated by the active distracting coping strategies. When the active distracting coping strategies are increasingly used by the patients, the association of depression with purpose in life is negative, which means that in case if the patients are using the active distracting coping strategies the depression increases and purpose in life decreases.

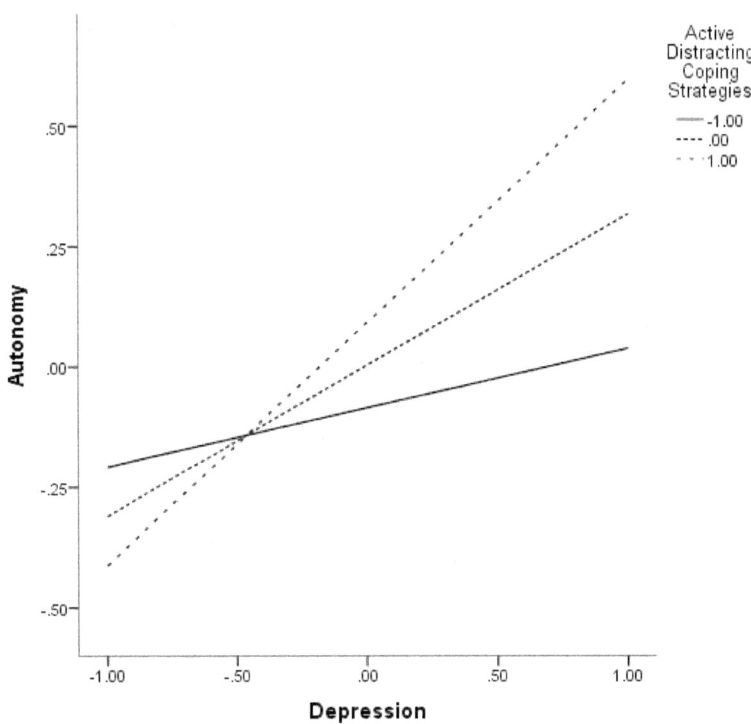

Figure 13. Active Distracting coping strategies as a moderator between autonomy and depression

The correlation of depression with autonomy is moderated by the active distracting coping strategies. When the active distracting coping strategies are increasingly used by the patients, the depression and autonomy is positively associated, which means that in case if the patients are using the active distracting coping strategies the depression increases and autonomy also increases.

Table 51

Moderating Effect of Avoidance-Focused Coping strategies on Relationship of Depression with Environmental Mastery, Self-Acceptance, Positive Relations, Purpose In Life, Autonomy and Personal Growth (n = 500)

Variables	Environmental Mastery		Self-acceptance		Positive relation		Purpose in life		Personal growth		Autonomy	
	ΔR^2	β	ΔR^2	β	ΔR^2	β	ΔR^2	β	ΔR^2	β	ΔR^2	β
Step 1												
Depression		-.42**		-.37**		-.43**		-.42*		-.44**		.36**
Avoidance-Focused coping		.06		-.24		.11		.23**		-.07		.24**
Step 2	.01		.00		.01		.01		.01		.01	
Depression * Avoidance-Focused coping		-.20**		-.07		-.19*		-.16*		-.15*		.15
R^2	.21		.14		.23		.25		.20		.14	

$** p < .01, * p < .05.$

Table 51 illustrates moderation analysis for avoidance focused coping strategies in the relationship between depression and Psychological well-being (environmental mastery, positive relations, purpose in life and personal growth). Avoidance focused coping strategies are acting as a moderator for the relationship of depression with environmental mastery, positive relations, purpose in life and personal growth. Moderation analysis for active coping strategies in the relationship between depression and autonomy doesn't occur. These added additional 1% variance is explained by the relationship (environmental mastery and depression) which is moderated by avoidance focused coping strategies. It also added additional 1% variance is explained by the relationship (positive relations with others and depression) which is moderated by avoidance focused coping strategies. It also added additional 1% variance is explained by the relationship (purpose in life and depression) which is moderated by avoidance focused coping strategies. Furthermore, it also added additional 1% variance is explained by the relationship (personal growth and depression) which is moderated by avoidance focused coping strategies. The moderating effect is further explained through mod graphs.

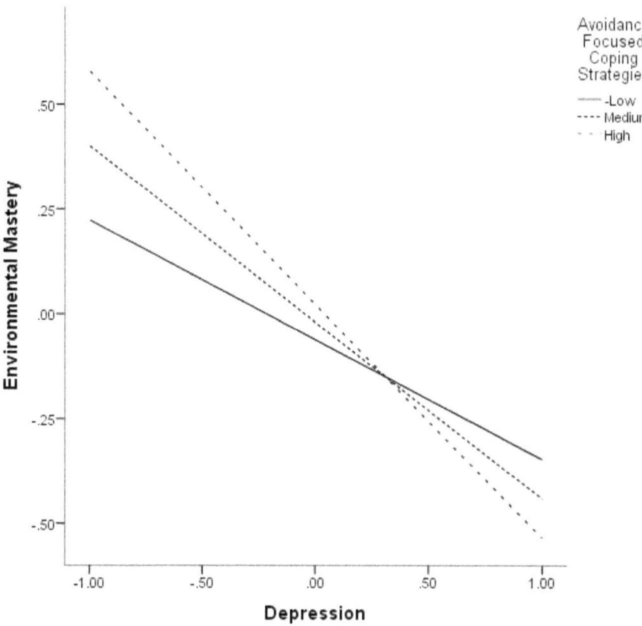

Figure 14. Avoidance focused coping strategies as a moderator between environmental mastery and depression

The association between the depression and environmental mastery is moderated by the avoidance focused coping strategies. When the avoidance focused coping strategies are increasingly used by the patients, the association of depression with environmental mastery is negative, which means that in case if the patients are using the avoidance focused coping strategies the depression increases and environmental mastery decreases.

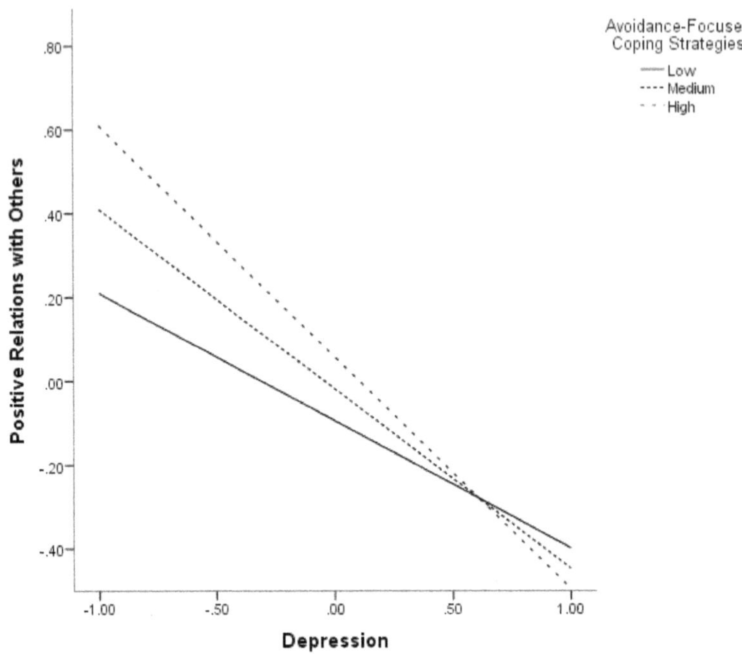

Figure 15. Avoidance focused coping strategies as a moderator between positive relations with others and depression

The correlation of depression with positive relations with others is moderated by the avoidance focused coping strategies. When the avoidance focused coping strategies are increasingly used by the patients, the association of depression with positive relations with others is negative, which means that in case if the patients are using the avoidance focused coping strategies the depression increases and positive relations with others decreases.

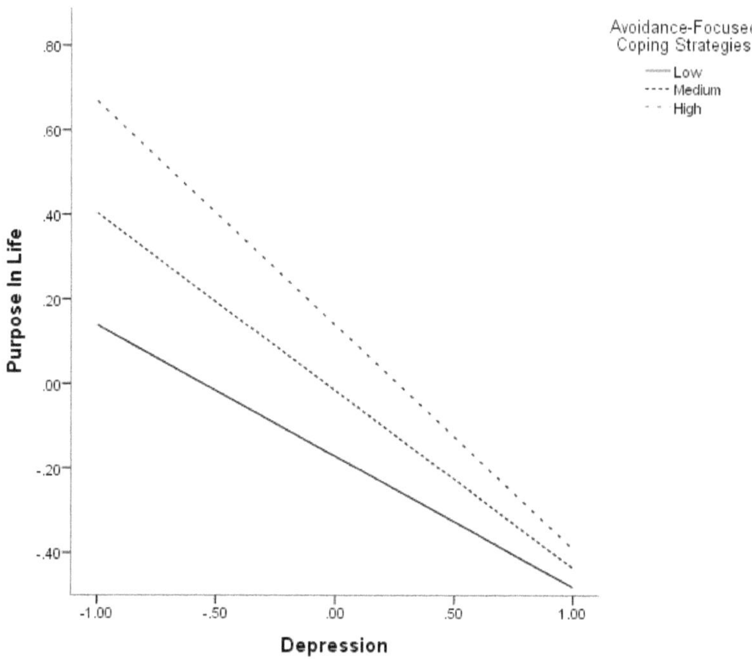

Figure 16. Avoidance focused coping strategies as a moderator between purpose in life and depression

The correlation of depression with purpose in life is moderated by the avoidance focused coping strategies. When the avoidance focused coping strategies are increasingly used by the patients, the association of depression with purpose in life is negative, which means that in case if the patients are using the avoidance focused coping strategies the depression increases and purpose in life decreases.

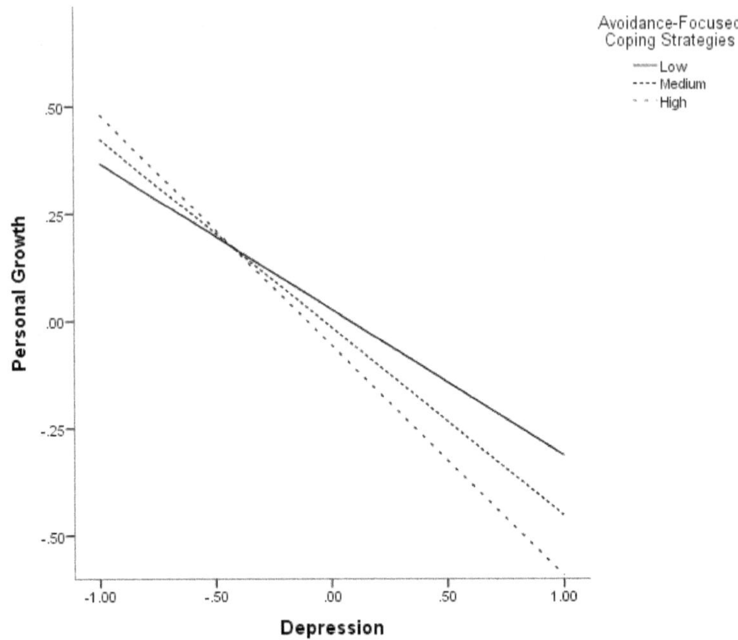

Figure 17. Avoidance focused coping strategies as a moderator between personal growth and depression

The correlation of depression with personal growth is moderated by the avoidance focused coping strategies. When the avoidance focused coping strategies are increasingly used by the patients, the association with depression with personal growth is negative, which means that in case if the patients are using the avoidance focused coping strategies the depression increases and personal growth decreases.

Table 52

Moderating Effect of Religious-Focused Coping strategies on Relationship of Depression with Environmental Mastery, Self-Acceptance, Positive Relations, Purpose In Life, Autonomy and Personal Growth (n = 500)

Variables	Environmental Mastery		Self-acceptance		Positive relation		Purpose in life		Personal growth		Autonomy	
	ΔR^2	β	ΔR^2	β	ΔR^2	β	ΔR^2	β	ΔR^2	β	ΔR^2	β
Step 1												
Depression		-.40**		-.34**		-.40**		-.43		-.41**		.36**
Religious-Focused coping		-.63		-.09		-.07		.02		.12**		.00
Step 2	.01		.00		.02		.00		.01		.00	
Depression * Religious-Focused coping		-.10*		-.03		-.14**		-.04		-.10*		-.03
R^2	.21		.04		.23		.20		.23		.12	

** $p < .01$, * $p < .05$.

Table 52 illustrates moderation analysis for religious focused coping strategies in the relationship between depression and Psychological well-being (environmental mastery, positive relations, and personal growth). Religious focused coping strategies are acting as a moderator for the relationship of depression with environmental mastery, positive relations and personal growth. Moderation analysis for Religious focused coping strategies in the relationship between depression and autonomy doesn't occur. These added additional 1% variance is explained by the relationship (environmental mastery and depression) which is moderated by Religious focused coping strategies. It also added additional 2% variance is explained by the relationship (positive relations with others and depression) which is moderated by Religious focused coping strategies. Furthermore, it also added additional 1% variance is explained by the relationship (personal growth and depression) which is moderated by Religious focused coping strategies. The moderating effect is further explained through mod graphs.

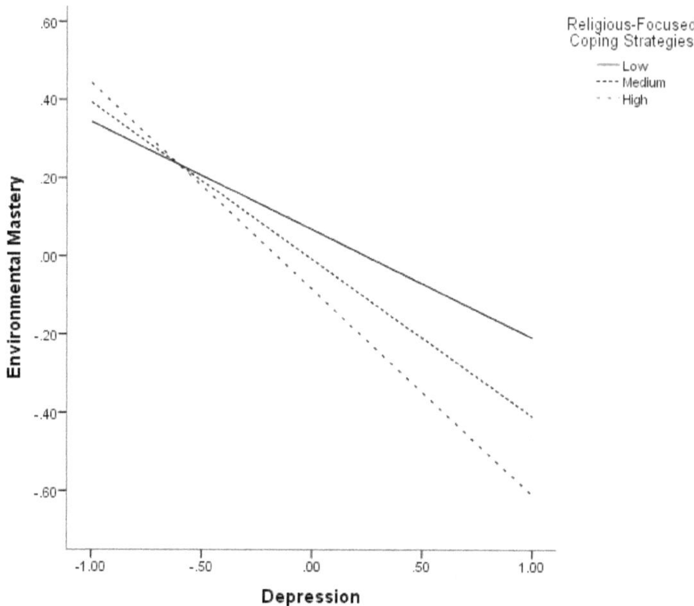

Figure 18. Religious focused coping strategies as a moderator between environmental mastery and depression

The association between the depression and environmental mastery is moderated by the religious focused coping strategies. When the religious focused coping strategies are increasingly used by the patients, the relationship between depression and environmental mastery is negative, which means that in case if the patients are using the religious focused coping strategies the depression increases and environmental mastery decreases.

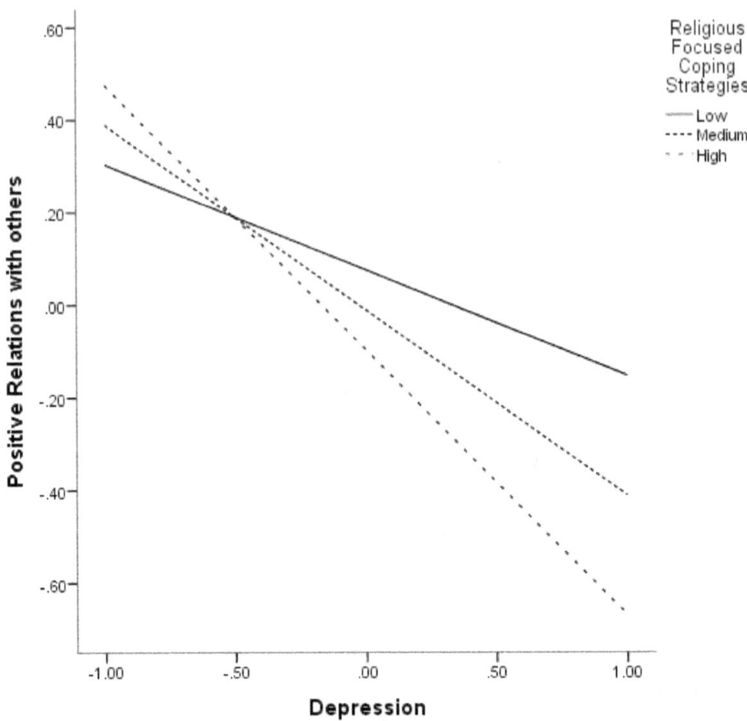

Figure 19. Religious focused coping strategies as a moderator between positive relations with others and depression

The association between the depression and positive relations with others is moderated by the religious focused coping strategies. When the religious focused coping strategies are increasingly used by the patients, the relationship between depression and positive relations with others is negative, which means that in case if the patients are using the religious focused coping strategies the depression increases and positive relations with others decreases.

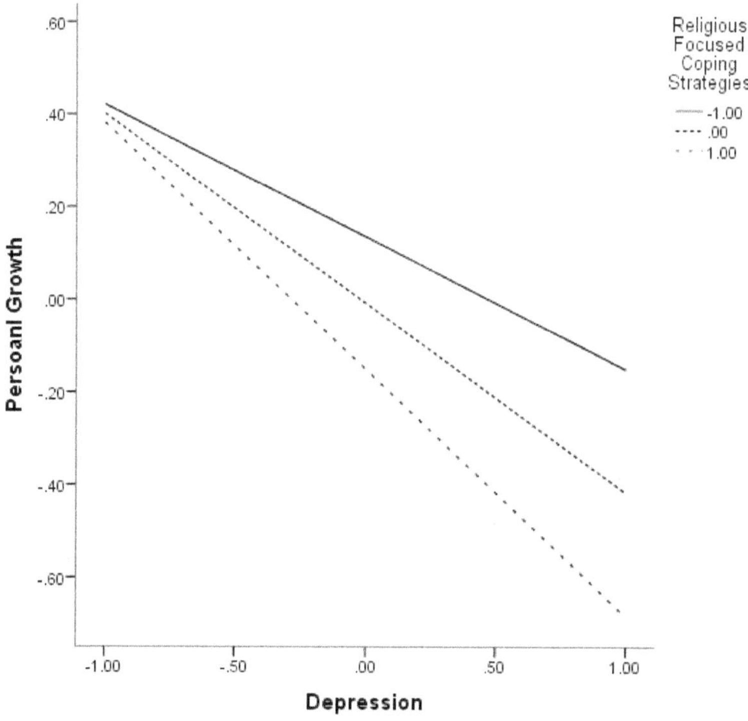

Figure 20. Religious focused coping strategies as a moderator between personal growth and depression

The correlation of depression with personal growth is moderated by the religious focused coping strategies. When the religious focused coping strategies are increasingly used by the patients, the relationship between depression and personal growth is negative, which means that in case if the patients are using the religious focused coping strategies the depression increases and personal growth decreases.

Table 53

Moderating Effect of Active Focused Coping Strategies on Relationship of Depression with Social Relationships (n = 500)

	Social relationships	
Variables	$\triangle R^2$	β
Step 1		
Depression		2.10
Active focused coping		9.16
Step 2	.00	
Depression * Active focused coping		.92
R^2	.36***	

***$p < .001$, ** $p < .01$, * $p < .05$.

Table 54 illustrates moderation analysis for active coping strategies in the relationship between anger and social relationships (quality of life). Active focused coping strategies are not acting as a moderator for the relationship of depression with social relationships.

Table 54

Moderating Effect of Active Distracting Coping Strategies on Relationship of Depression with Physical Health, Psychological Health, Social Relationships and Environment (n = 500)

	Social relationships	
Variables	$\triangle R^2$	β
Step 1		
Depression		.66
Active distracting coping		2.57***
Step 2	.015**	
Depression * Active distracting coping		1.36**
R^2	.07***	

***$p < .001$, ** $p < .01$, * $p < .05$.

Table 55 illustrates moderation analysis for active distracting coping strategies in the relationship between depression and Social relationships. Active distracting coping strategies are acting as a moderator for the relationship of depression with social relationships. It added the additional 15% of variance is explained by the relationship (depression and social relationships) which is moderated by active distracting coping strategies.

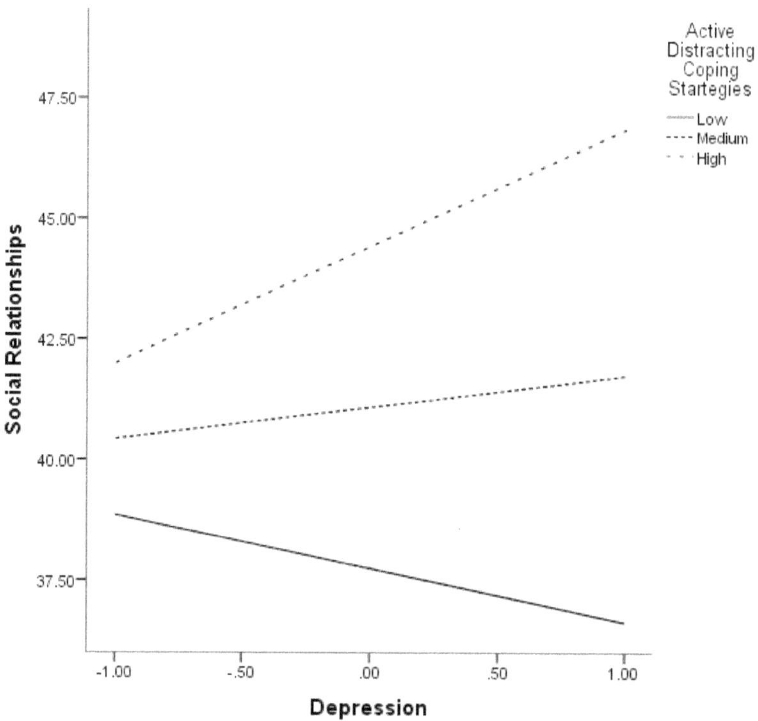

Figure 21. Active distracting coping strategies as a moderator between social relationships and depression

The association between the depression and social relationships is moderated by the active distracting coping strategies. When the active distracting coping strategies are increasingly used by the patients, the relationship between depression and social relationships is positive, which means that in case if the patients are using the active distracting coping strategies the depression increases and personal social relationships increase.

Table 55

Moderating Effect of Avoidance Focused Coping Strategies on Relationship of Depression with Social Relationships (n = 500)

	Social relationships	
Variables	ΔR^2	β
Step 1		
Depression		1.62**
Avoidance focused coping		9.21***
Step 2	.04***	
Depression * Avoidance focused coping		5.33***
R^2	.13***	

***p < .001, ** p < .01, * p < .05.

Table 55 illustrates moderation analysis for avoidance focused coping strategies in the relationship between depression and Social relationships. Active distracting coping strategies are acting as a moderator for the relationship of depression with social relationships. It added the additional 4% of variance is explained by the relationship (depression and social relationships) which is moderated by avoidance focused coping strategies.

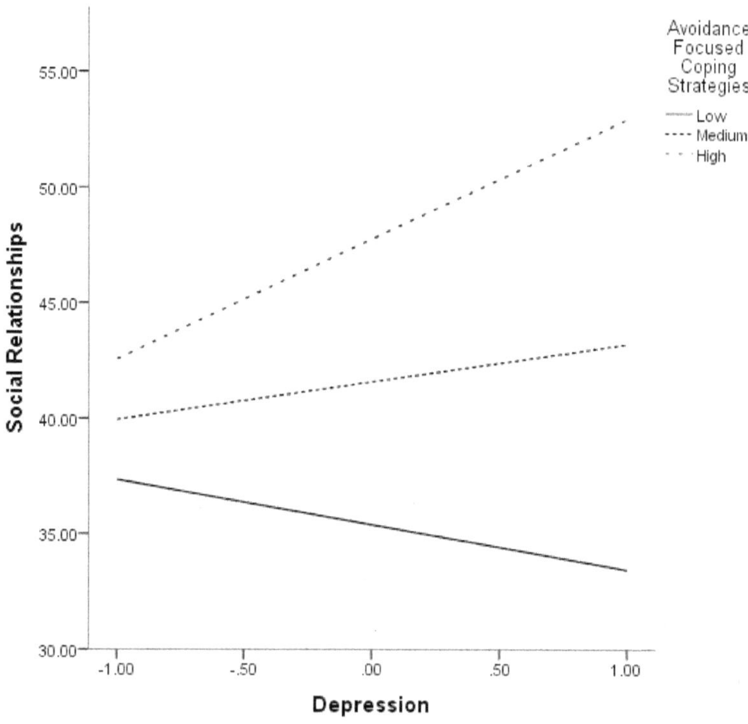

Figure 22. Avoidance focused coping strategies as a moderator between social relationships and depression

The correlation of depression with social relationships is moderated by the avoidance focused coping strategies. When the avoidance focused coping strategies are increasingly used by the patients, the relationship between depression and social relationships is positive, which means that in case if the patients are using the avoidance focused coping strategies the depression increases and social relationships increase.

Table 56

Moderating Effect of Religious Focused Coping Strategies on Relationship of Depression with Social Relationships (n = 500)

Variables	Social relationships	
	$\triangle R^2$	β
Step 1		
Depression		1.06
Religious focused coping		4.98***
Step 2	.00	
Depression * Religious focused coping		.646
R^2	.41***	

***$p < .001$, ** $p < .01$, * $p < .05$.

Table 56 illustrates moderation analysis for religious focused coping strategies in the relationship between depression and Social relationships. Religious focused coping strategies are not acting as a moderator for the relationship of depression with social relationships.

Table 57

Moderating Effect of tangible Support on Relationship of Depression with Social Relationships (n = 500)

Variables	Social relationships	
	$\triangle R^2$	β
Step 1		
Depression		-.21
Tangible Support		1.49***
Step 2	.07***	
Depression * Tangible Support		1.22***
R^2	.22***	

***$p < .001$, ** $p < .01$, * $p < .05$.

Table 57 illustrates moderation analysis for Tangible Support in the relationship between depression and Social relationships. Tangible Support is acting as a moderator for the relationship of depression with social relationships. The additional 7% of the variance is explained by the relationship (self-acceptance and depression) which is moderated by the tangible support.

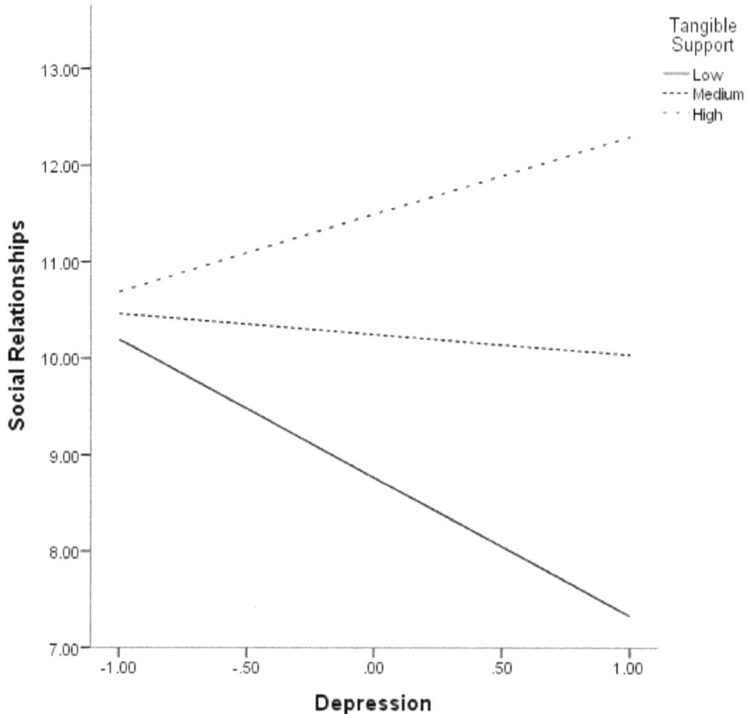

Figure 23. Tangible support as a moderator between social relationships and depression

The correlation of depression with social relationships is moderated by the Tangible Support. When the Tangible Support is increasingly used by the patients, the relationship between depression and social relationships is negative, which means that in case if the patients are using the Tangible Support the depression increases and social relationships decreases. But as according to scoring if the scores are low in support it indicates that the support is high and if scored are high the support is low. So if the person is having less tangible support the relationship between the depression and social relationship is negative and depression is high and social relationships are low.

Table 58

Moderating Effect of emotional Support on Relationship of Depression with Social Relationships (n = 500)

	Social relationships	
Variables	ΔR^2	β
Step 1		
Depression		.42**
Emotional Support		1.66***
Step 2	.001	
Depression * Emotional Support		.09
R^2	.46***	

*** $p < .001$, ** $p < .01$, * $p < .05$.

Table 58 illustrates moderation analysis for Emotional Support in the relationship between depression and Social relationships. Emotional Support is not acting as a moderator for the relationship of depression with social relationships.

Table 59

Moderating Effect of Esteem Support on Relationship of Depression with Social Relationships (n = 500)

	Social relationships	
Variables	ΔR^2	β
Step 1		
Depression		.37*
Esteem Support		1.91***
Step 2	.001	
Depression * Esteem Support		.16
R^2	.53***	

*** $p < .001$, ** $p < .01$, * $p < .05$.

Table 59 illustrates moderation analysis for Esteem Support in the relationship between depression and Social relationships. Esteem Support is not acting as a moderator for the relationship of depression with social relationships.

Table 60

Moderating Effect of Social Network Support on Relationship of Depression with Social Relationships (n = 500)

	Social relationships	
Variables	ΔR^2	β
Step 1		
Depression		.33**
Social network Support		2.19***
Step 2	.01*	
Depression		.34*
* Social network Support		
R^2	.61***	

***$p < .001$, ** $p < .01$, * $p < .05$.

Table 60 illustrates moderation analysis for Social Network Support in the relationship between depression and Social relationships. Social Network Support is acting as a moderator for the relationship of depression with social relationships. The additional 1% of the variance is explained by the relationship (self-acceptance and depression) which is moderated by the Social Network Support.

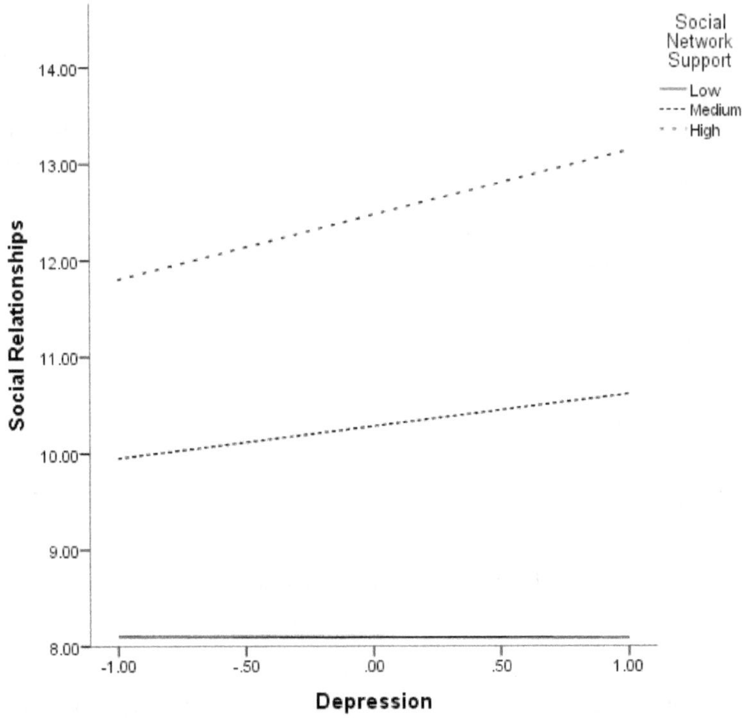

Figure 24. Social network support as a moderator between social relationships and depression

The correlation between the depression with social relationships is moderated by the Social Network Support. When the Social Network Support is increasingly used by the patients, the relationship between depression and social relationships is positive, which means that in case if the patients are using the Social Network Support the depression increases and social relationships also increase.

Table 61

Moderating Effect of Informational Support on Relationship of Depression with Environmental Mastery, Self-Acceptance, Positive Relations, Purpose in Life, Autonomy and Personal Growth (n = 500)

Variables	Environmental Mastery		Self-acceptance		Positive relation		Purpose in life		Personal growth		Autonomy	
	ΔR^2	β	ΔR^2	β	ΔR^2	β	ΔR^2	β	ΔR^2	β	ΔR^2	β
Step 1												
Depression		-.39***		-.27***		-.46***		-.41***		-.44***		.26***
Informational Support		-.28***		-3.65**		-.19***		-.33***		-.25***		.19***
Step 2	.00		.027**		.01*		.00		.00		.03***	
Depression * Informational Support		-.07		-.19		.09*		-.06		.05		.23***
R²	.27***		.17***		.24***		.31***		.26***		.19***	

** $p < .01$, * $p < .05$.

Table 61 illustrates moderation analysis for informational support in the relationship between depression and Psychological well-being (environmental mastery, positive relations, and personal growth). Informational support is acting as a moderator for the relationship of depression with self-acceptance, positive relations with others and autonomy. Moderation analyses for Informational support in the relationship of depression with environmental mastery, purpose in life and personal growth doesn't occur. These added additional 2.7% variance is explained by the relationship (self-acceptance and depression) which is moderated by informational support. It also added additional 1% variance is explained by the relationship (positive relations with others and depression) which is moderated by Religious focused coping strategies. Furthermore, it also added additional 3% variance is explained by the relationship (autonomy and depression) which is moderated by informational support. The moderating effect is further explained through mod graphs.

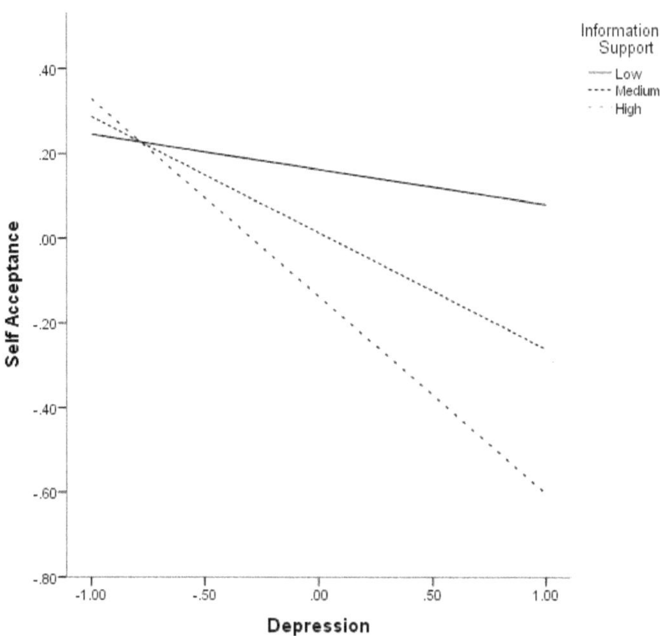

Figure 25. Informational support as a moderator between self-acceptance and depression

The correlation of depression with self-acceptance is moderated by the Informational support. When the Informational support is increasingly used by the patients, the relationship between depression and self-acceptance is negative, which means that in case if the patients are using the Informational support the depression increases and self-acceptance decreases.

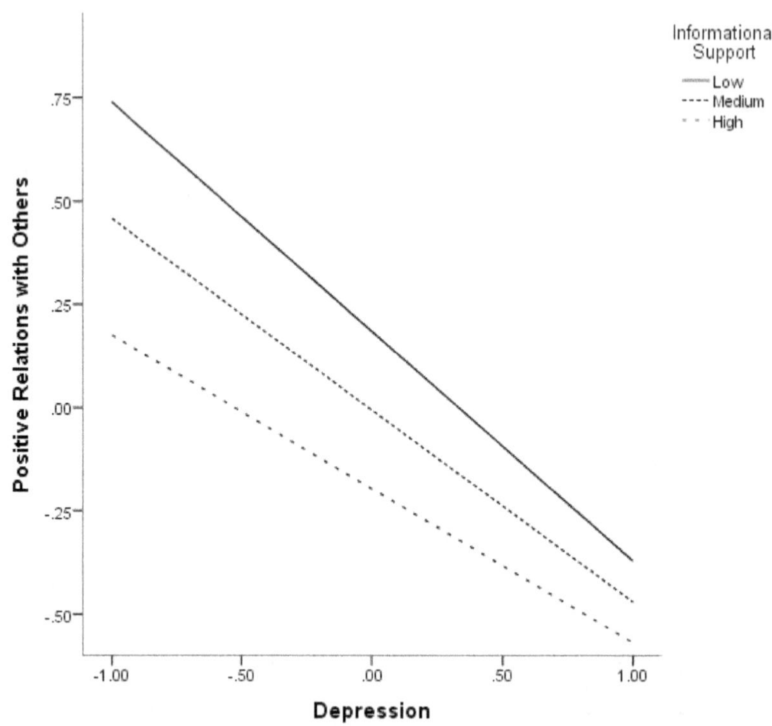

Figure 26. Informational support as a moderator between positive relationships with others and depression

The correlation of depression with positive relations with others is moderated by the Informational support. When the Informational support is increasingly used by the patients, the relationship between depression and positive relations with others is negative, which means that in case if the patients are using the Informational support the depression increases and positive relations with others decreases.

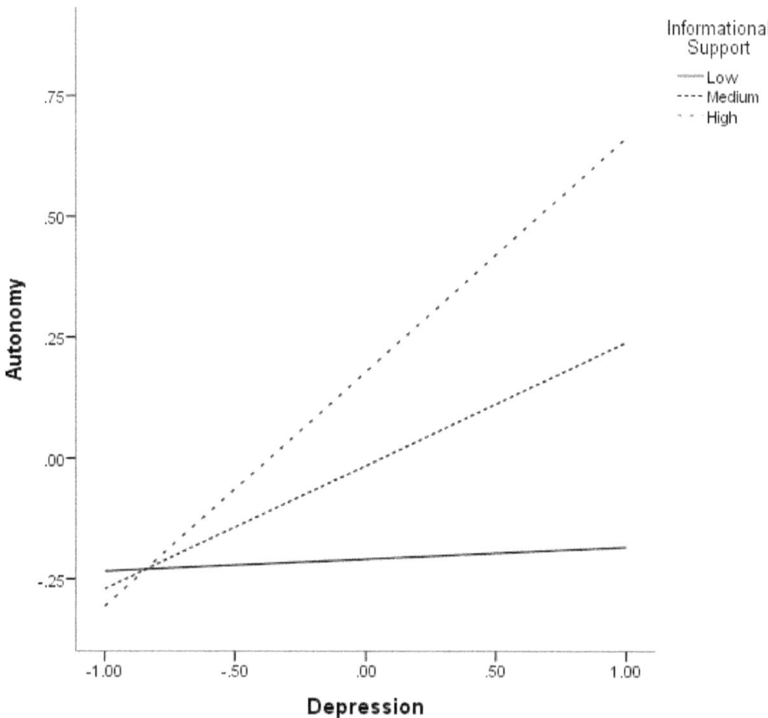

Figure 27. Informational support as a moderator between autonomy and depression

The correlation of depression with autonomy is moderated by the Informational support. When the Informational support is increasingly used by the patients, the relationship between depression and autonomy is positive, which means that in case if the patients are using the Informational support the depression increases and autonomy also increase.

Table 62

Moderating Effect of informational Support on Relationship of Depression with Social Relationships (n = 500)

Variables	Social relationships	
	ΔR^2	β
Step 1		
Depression		-.28
Informational Support		4.76***
Step 2	.02**	
Depression * Informational Support		2.55**
R^2	.12***	

$***p < .001, ** p < .01, * p < .05.$

Table 62 illustrates moderation analysis for Informational Support in the relationship between depression and Social relationships. Informational Support is acting as a moderator for the relationship of depression with social relationships. The additional 2% of the variance is explained by the relationship (self-acceptance and depression) which is moderated by the tangible support.

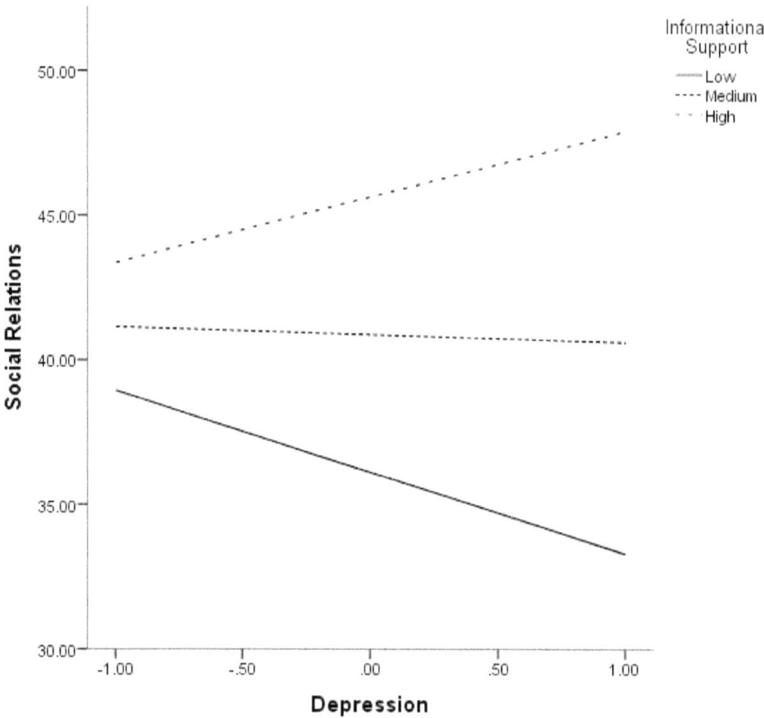

Figure 28. Informational support as a moderator between social relations and depression

The correlation of depression with social relations is moderated by the Informational support. When the Informational support is increasingly used by the patients, the relationship between depression and self-acceptance is positive, which means that in case if the patients are using the Informational support the depression increases and social relations also increase.

Table 63

Moderating Effect of Tangible Support on Relationship of Depression with Environmental Mastery, Self-Acceptance, Positive Relations, Purpose In Life, Autonomy and Personal Growth (n = 500)

Variables	Environmental Mastery		Self-acceptance		Positive relation		Purpose in life		Personal growth		Autonomy	
	ΔR^2	β	ΔR^2	β	ΔR^2	β	ΔR^2	β	ΔR^2	β	ΔR^2	β
Step 1												
Depression		-.36***		-.27***		-.41***		-.42***		-.38***		.30***
Tangible Support		-.32***		-.19***		-.25***		-.19***		-.30***		-.13***
Step 2	.03***		.03***		.01*		.00		.01**		.01*	
Depression * Tangible Support		-.21***		-.22***		-.10*		-.07		-.15**		.13*
R²	.31***		.18***		.27***		.24***		.29***		.38***	

** *p* < .01, * *p* < .05.

156

Table 63 illustrates the moderation analysis for tangible support in the relationship between depression and Psychological well-being (environmental mastery, positive relations, and personal growth). Tangible support is acting as a moderator for the relationship of depression with environmental mastery, self-acceptance, positive relations with others, personal growth and autonomy. Moderation analyses for tangible support in the relationship between depression and purpose in life doesn't occur. These added additional 3% of the variance is explained by the relationship (environmental mastery and depression) which is moderated by tangible support.   The additional 3% of the variance is explained by the relationship (self-acceptance and depression) which is moderated by the tangible support. It also added additional 1% variance is explained by the relationship (positive relations with others and depression) which is moderated by tangible support. Furthermore, it also added additional 1% variance is explained by the relationship (autonomy and depression) which is moderated by informational support. The moderating effect is further explained through mod graphs.

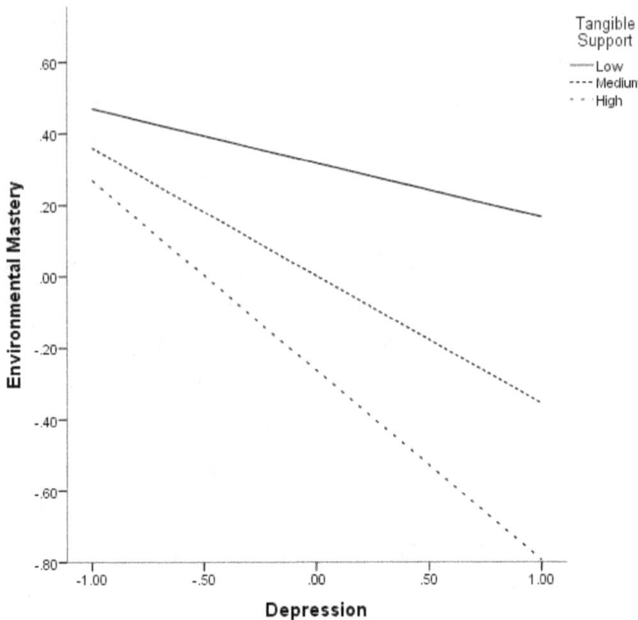

Figure 29. Tangible support as a moderator between environmental mastery and depression

The correlation of depression with environmental mastery is moderated by the tangible support. When the tangible support is increasingly used by the patients, the relationship between depression and environmental mastery is negative, which means that in case if the patients are using the tangible support the depression increases and environmental mastery decreases.

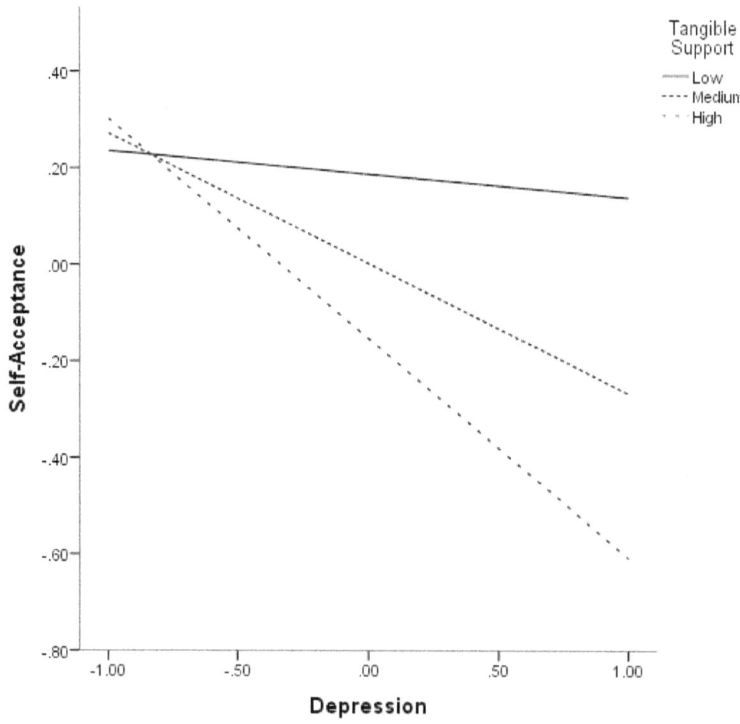

Figure 30. Tangible support as a moderator between self-acceptance and depression

The correlation between the depression with self-acceptance is moderated by the tangible support. When the tangible support is increasingly used by the patients, the relationship between depression and self-acceptance is negative, which means that in case if the patients are using the tangible support the depression increases and self-acceptance decreases.

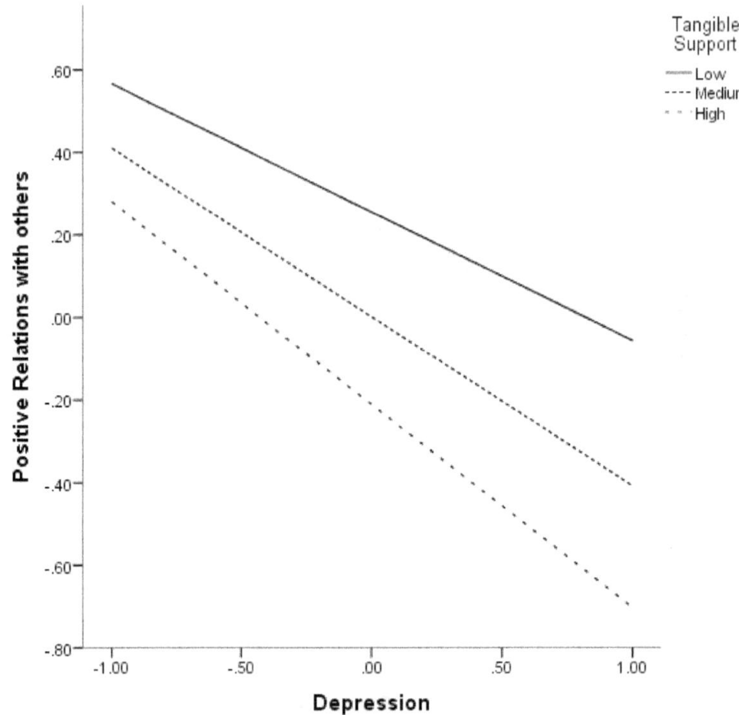

Figure 31. Tangible support as a moderator between positive relations with others and depression

The correlation between the depression with positive relations with others is moderated by the tangible support. When the tangible support is increasingly used by the patients, the relationship between depression and positive relations with others is negative, which means that in case if the patients are using the tangible support the depression increases and positive relations with others decreases.

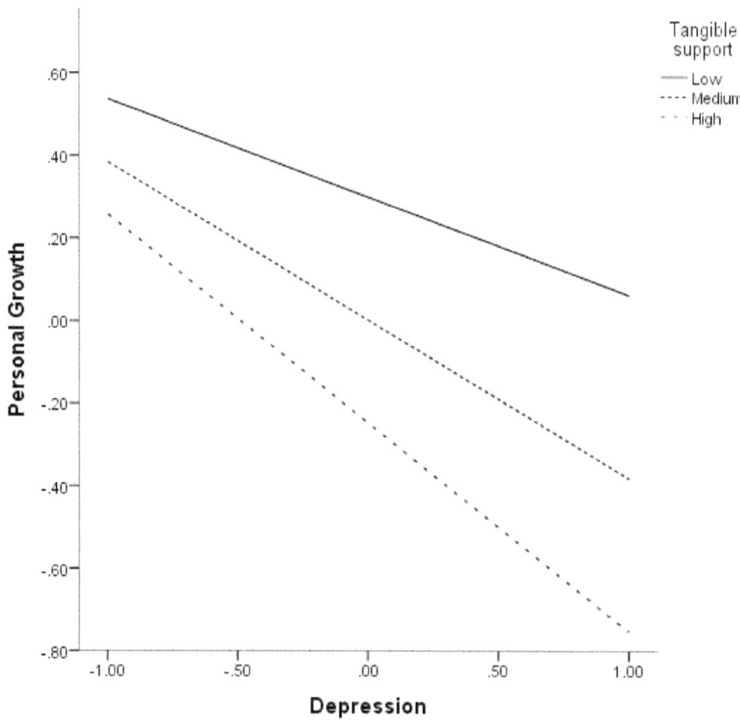

Figure 32. Tangible support as a moderator between personal growth and depression

The correlation of depression with personal growth is moderated by the tangible support. When the tangible support is increasingly used by the patients, the relationship between depression and personal growth is negative, which means that in case if the patients are using the tangible support the depression increases and personal growth decreases.

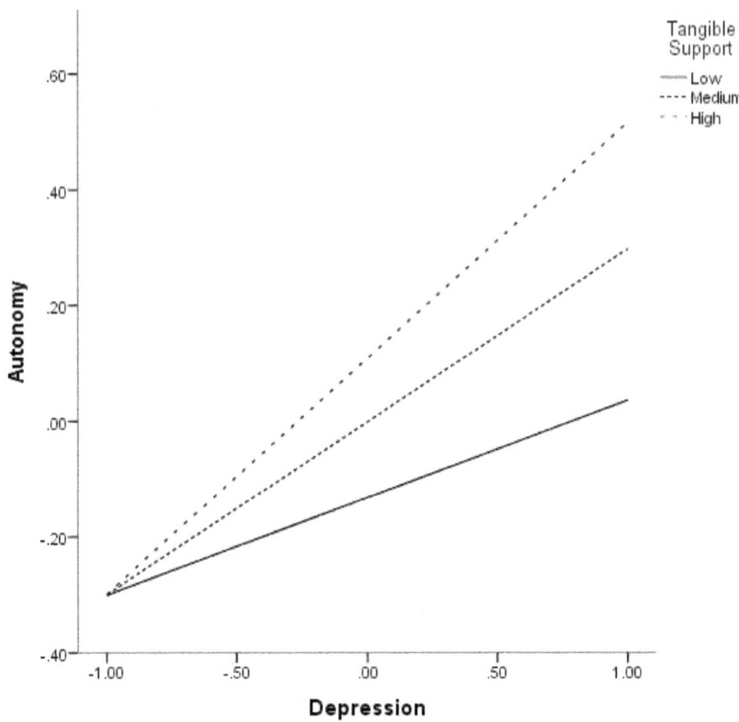

Figure 33. Tangible support as a moderator between autonomy and depression

The correlation between the depression with autonomy is moderated by the tangible support. When the tangible support is increasingly used by the patients, the relationship between depression and personal growth is positive, which means that in case if the patients are using the tangible support the depression increases and autonomy decreases..

Table 64

Moderating Effect of Esteem Support on Relationship of Depression with Environmental Mastery, Self-Acceptance, Positive Relations, Purpose In Life, Autonomy and Personal Growth (n = 500)

Variables	Environmental Mastery ΔR^2	β	Self-acceptance ΔR^2	β	Positive relation ΔR^2	β	Purpose in life ΔR^2	β	Personal growth ΔR^2	β	Autonomy ΔR^2	β
Step 1												
Depression		-.42***		-.31***		-.44***		-.43***		-.45***		.33***
Esteem Support		-.18***		-.03		-.07		-.04		-.22***		.10*
Step 2	.03***		-.26***		.01*		.02**		.00		.42***	
Depression * Esteem Support		-.20***		-.26***		-.10*		-.16**		-.07		.19***
R^2	.28***		.43***		.22***		.23***		.50***		.03***	

** $p < .01$, * $p < .05$.

Table 64 illustrates moderation analysis for esteem support in the relationship between depression and Psychological well-being (environmental mastery, self-acceptance, positive relations with others, purpose in life and autonomy). Esteem support is acting as a moderator for the relationship of depression with environmental mastery, self-acceptance, positive relations with others, purpose in life and autonomy. Moderation analyses for esteem support in the relationship between depressions with purpose in life doesn't occur. This added additional 3% of the variance is explained by the relationship (environmental mastery and depression) which is moderated by emotional support. The additional 26% of the variance is explained by the relationship (self-acceptance and depression) which is moderated by the esteem support. It also added additional 1% variance is explained by the relationship (positive relations with others and depression) which is moderated by esteem support. It also added additional 2% variance is explained by the relationship (purpose in life and depression) which is moderated by esteem support. Furthermore, it also added additional 3% variance is explained by the relationship (autonomy and depression) which is moderated by emotional support. The moderating effect is further explained through mod graphs.

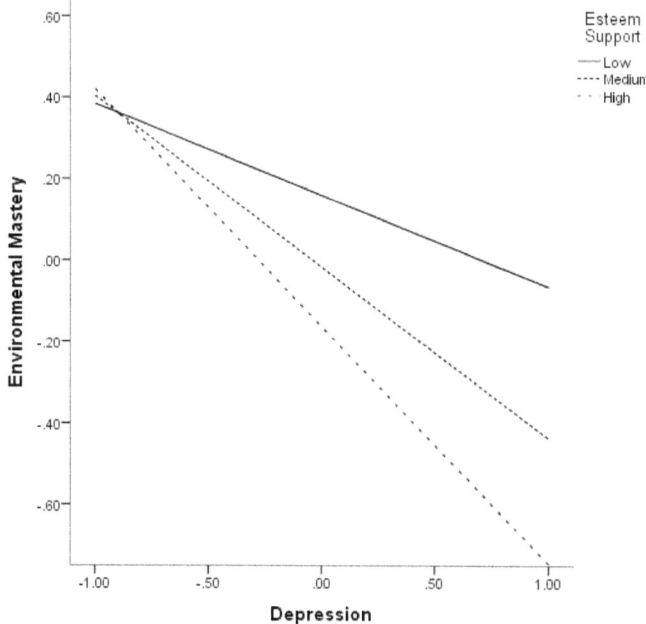

Figure 34. Esteem support as a moderator between environmental mastery and depression

The correlation between the depression with environmental mastery is moderated by the esteem support. When the esteem support is increasingly used by the patients, the relationship between depression and environmental mastery is negative, which means that in case if the patients are using the esteem support the depression increases and environmental mastery decreases.

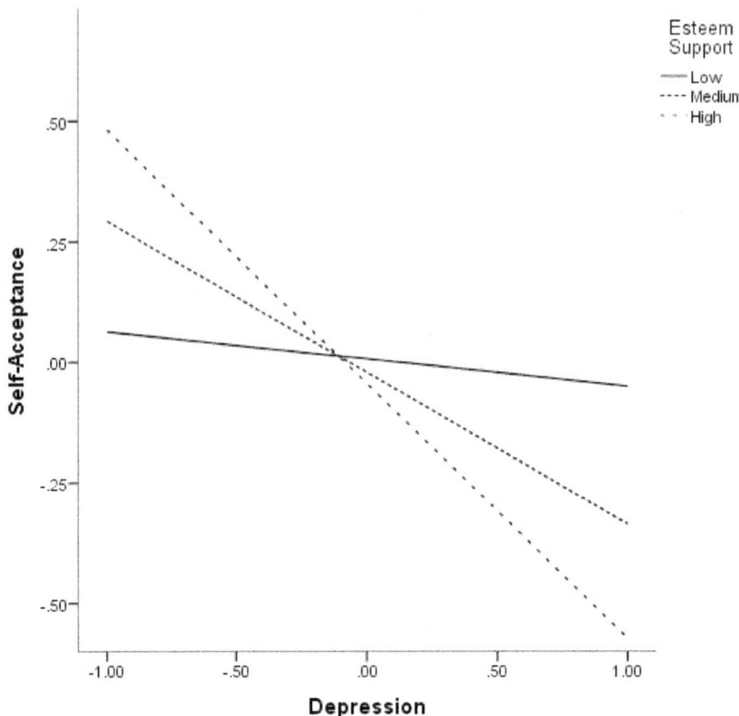

Figure 35. Esteem support as a moderator between self-acceptance and depression

The correlation of depression with self-acceptance is moderated by the esteem support. When the esteem support is increasingly used by the patients, the relationship between depression and self-acceptance is negative, which means that in case if the patients are using the esteem support the depression increases and self-acceptance decreases.

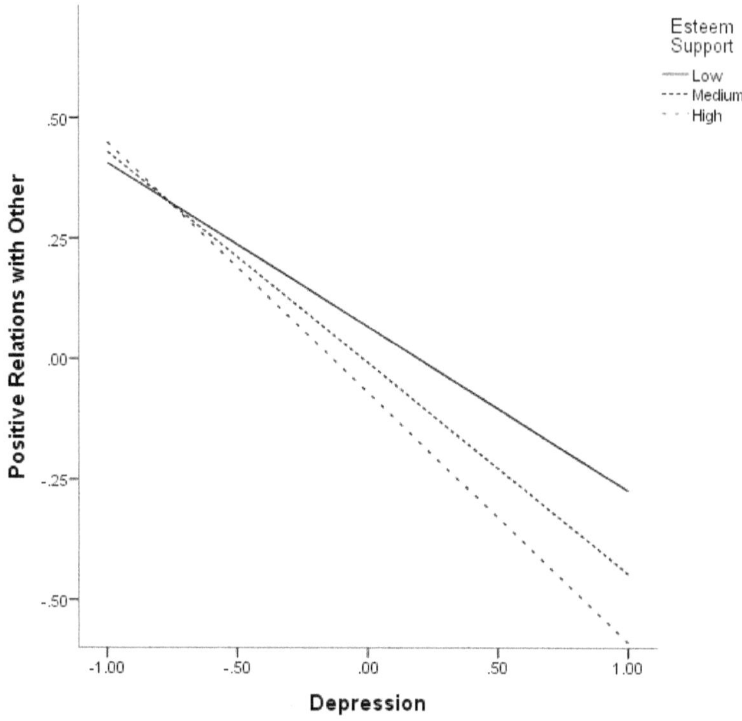

Figure 36. Esteem support as a moderator between positive relations with others and depression

    The correlation of depression with positive relations with others is moderated by the esteem support. When the esteem support is increasingly used by the patients, the relationship between depression and positive relations with others is negative, which means that in case if the patients are using the esteem support the depression increases and positive relations with others decreases.

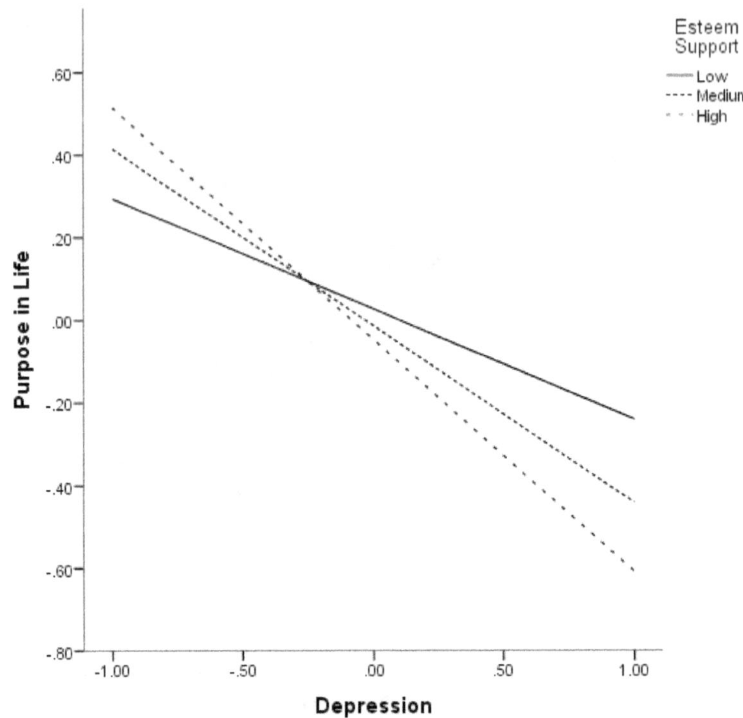

Figure 37. Esteem support as a moderator between purpose in life and depression

The correlation of depression with purpose in life is moderated by the esteem support. When the esteem support is increasingly used by the patients, the relationship between depression and purpose in life is negative, which means that in case if the patients are using the esteem support the depression increases and purpose in life decreases.

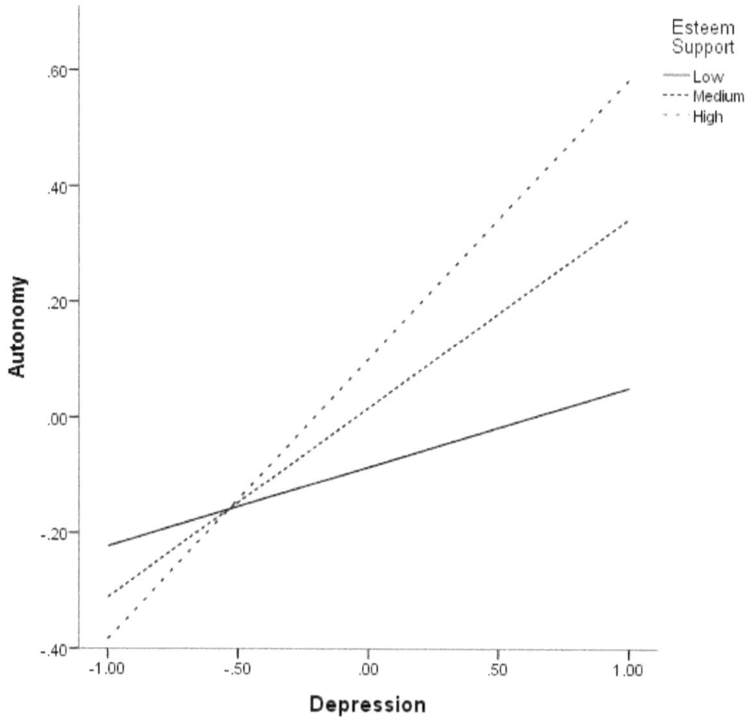

Figure 38. Esteem support as a moderator between autonomy and depression

The correlation between the depression with autonomy is moderated by the esteem support. When the esteem support is increasingly used by the patients, the relationship between depression and autonomy is positive, which means that in case if the patients are using the esteem support the depression increases and autonomy increase.

Table 65

Moderating Effect of Social Network Support on Relationship of Depression with Environmental Mastery, Self-Acceptance, Positive Relations, Purpose In Life, Autonomy and Personal Growth (n = 500)

Variables	Environmental Mastery		Self-acceptance		Positive relation		Purpose in life		Personal growth		Autonomy	
	ΔR^2	β	ΔR^2	β	ΔR^2	β	ΔR^2	β	ΔR^2	β	ΔR^2	β
Step 1												
Depression		-.43***		-.35***		-.45***		-.44***		-.45***		.35***
Social Network Support		-.14**		-2.97**		-.07		-.01		-.23***		.21***
Step 2	.03***		.03***		.00		.02**		.00		.02**	
Depression * Social Network Support		-.17***		-.17***		-.05		-.12**		-.03		.14**
R^2	.49***		.42***		.46***		.47***		.50***		.44***	

** $p < .01$, * $p < .05$.

Table 65 illustrates the moderation analysis for social network support in the relationship between depression and Psychological well-being (environmental mastery, self-acceptance, purpose in life and autonomy). Social network support is acting as a moderator for the relationship of depression with environmental mastery, self-acceptance, purpose in life and autonomy. Moderation analyses for esteem support in the relationship between depression with purpose in life doesn't occur. This added additional 3% of the variance is explained by the relationship (environmental mastery and depression) which is moderated by social network support. The additional 3% of the variance is explained by the relationship (self-acceptance and depression) which is moderated by the social network support. It also added additional 2% variance is explained by the relationship (purpose in life and depression) which is moderated by social network support. Furthermore, it also added additional 2% variance is explained by the relationship (autonomy and depression) which is moderated by social network support. The moderating effect is further explained through mod graphs.

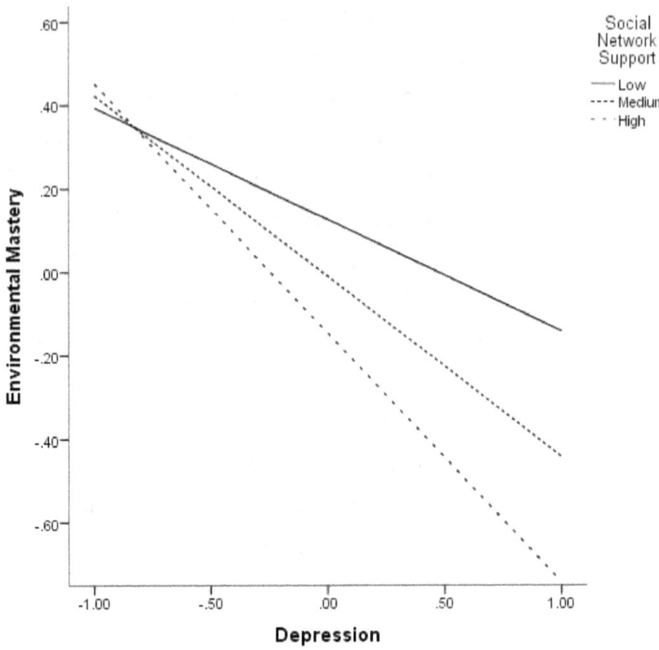

Figure 39. Social network support as a moderator between environmental mastery and depression

The correlation between the depression with environmental mastery is moderated by the social network support. When the social network support is increasingly used by the patients, the relationship between depression and environmental mastery is negative, which means that in case if the patients are using the social network support the depression increases and environmental mastery decreases.

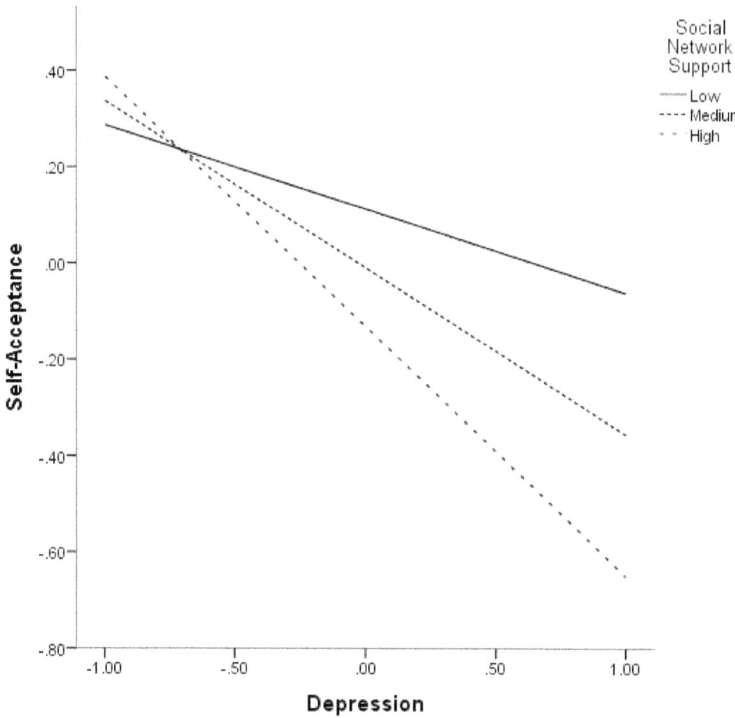

Figure 40. Social network support as a moderator between self-acceptance and depression

The correlation of depression with self-acceptance is moderated by the social network support. When the social network support is increasingly used by the patients, the relationship between depression and self-acceptance is negative, which means that in case if the patients are using the social network support the depression increases and self-acceptance decreases.

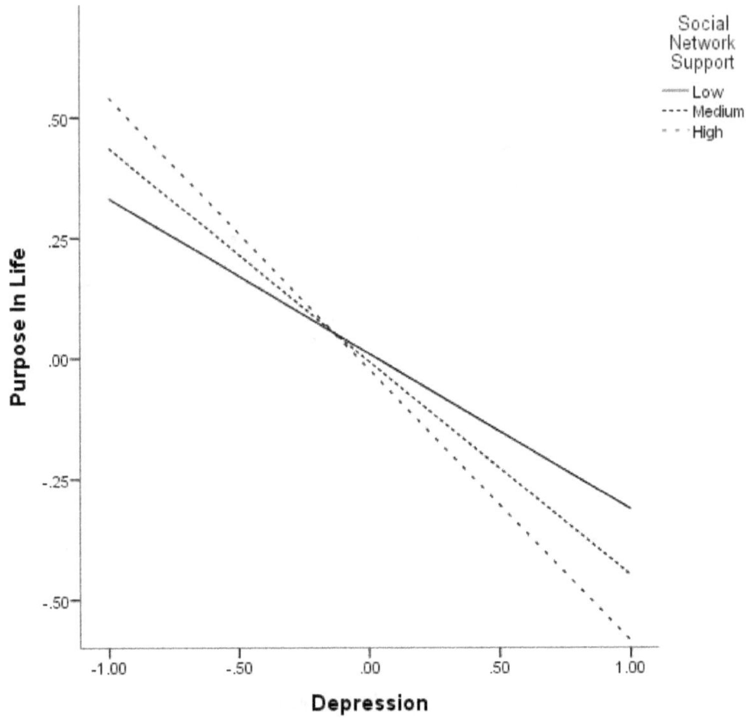

Figure 41. Social network support as a moderator between purpose in life and depression

The correlation of depression with purpose in life is moderated by the social network support. When the social network support is increasingly used by the patients, the relationship between depression and purpose in life is negative, which means that in case if the patients are using the social network support the depression increases and purpose in life decreases.

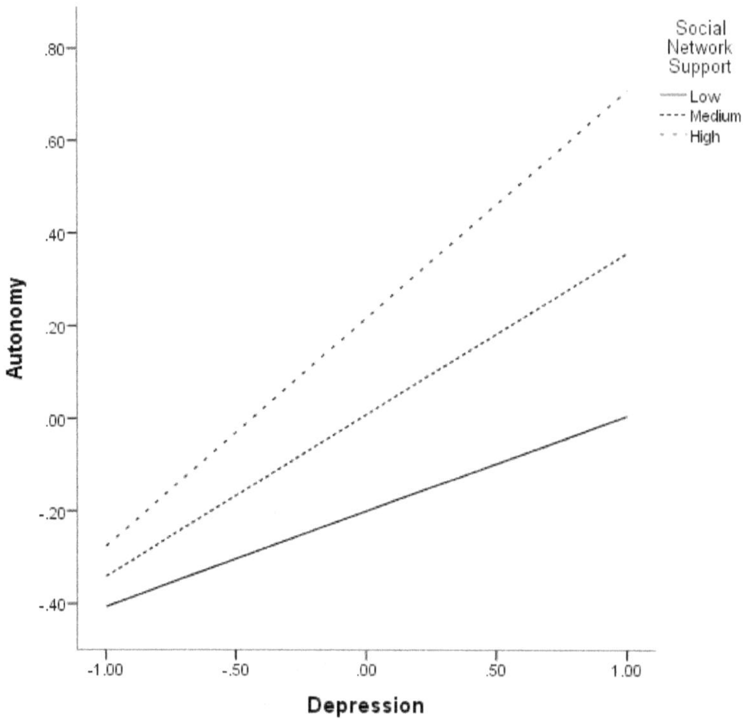

Figure 42. Social network support as a moderator between autonomy and depression

The correlation of depression with autonomy is moderated by the social network support. When the social network support is increasingly used by the patients, the relationship between depression and autonomy is positive, which means that in case if the patients are using the social network support the depression increases and purpose in life increase.

Table 66

Moderating Effect of Active focused coping strategies on Relationship of State Anger with Environmental Mastery and Personal Growth (n = 500)

Variables	Environmental Mastery		Personal growth	
	ΔR^2	β	ΔR^2	β
Step 1				
State Anger		-.28***		-.27***
Active Focused Coping Strategies		-.03		-.11*
Step 2	.09***		.04***	
State Anger				-.19***
* Active Focused Coping Strategies		-.27***		
R^2	.11***		.26***	

** $p < .01$, * $p < .05$.

Table 66 illustrates moderation analysis for active focused coping strategies in the relationship between State Anger and Psychological well-being (environmental mastery and personal growth). Active focused coping strategies are acting as a moderator for the relationship of state anger with environmental mastery and personal growth. This added additional 9% of the variance is explained by the relationship (environmental mastery and state anger) which is moderated by active focused coping strategies. The additional 4% of the variance is explained by the relationship (personal growth and state anger) which is moderated by the active focused coping strategies. The moderating effect is further explained through mod graphs.

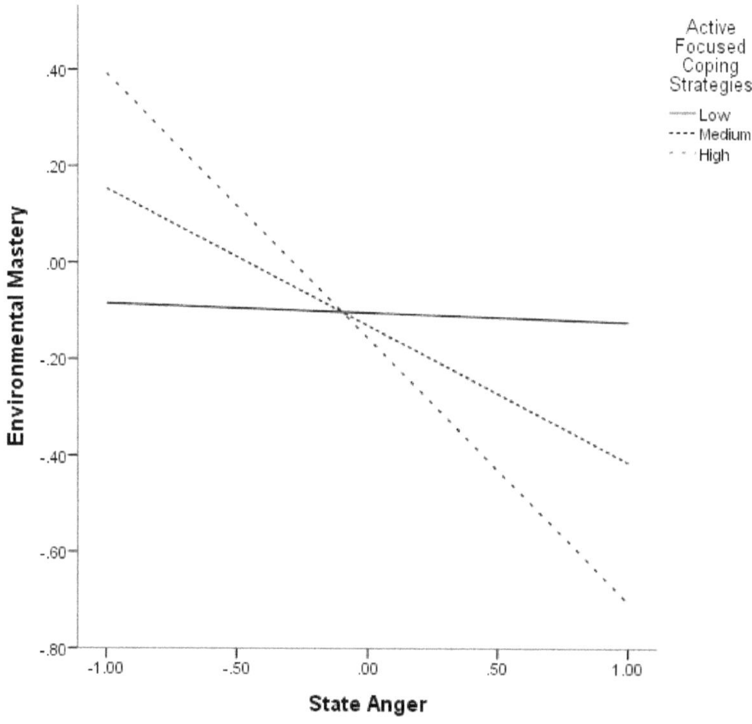

Figure 43. Active focused coping strategies as a moderator between environmental mastery and state anger

The correlation between the state anger with environmental mastery is moderated by the Active focused coping strategies. When the Active focused coping strategies is increasingly used by the patients, the relationship between state anger and environmental mastery is negative, which means that in case if the patients are using the Active focused coping strategies the state anger increases and environmental mastery decreases.

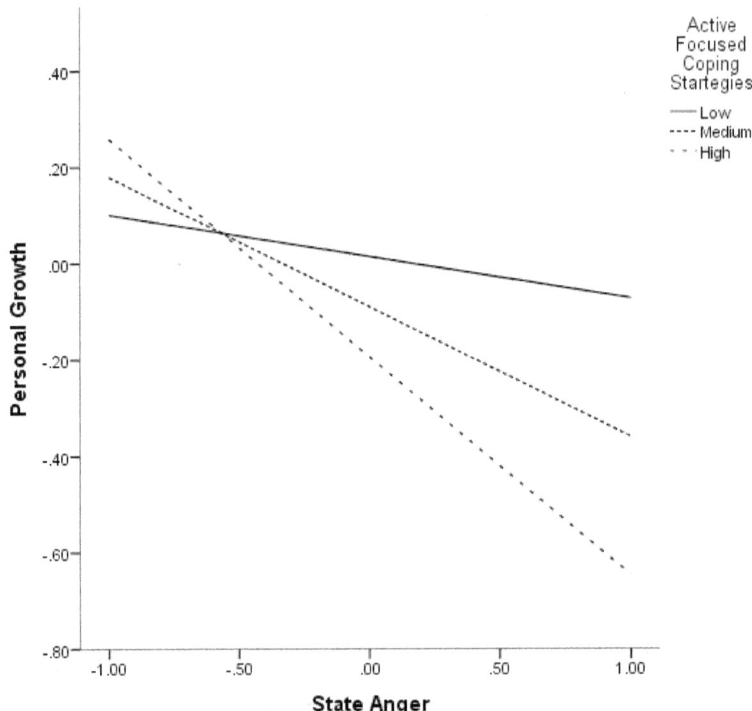

Figure 44. Active focused coping strategies as a moderator between personal growth and state anger

The correlation between the state anger with personal growth is moderated by the Active focused coping strategies. When the Active focused coping strategies is increasingly used by the patients, the relationship between state anger and personal growth is negative, which means that in case if the patients are using the Active focused coping strategies the state anger increases and personal growth decreases.

Table 67

Moderating Effect of Avoidance focused coping strategies on Relationship of State Anger with Environmental Mastery and Personal Growth (n = 500)

Variables	Environmental Mastery		Personal growth	
	$\triangle R^2$	β	$\triangle R^2$	β
Step 1				
State Anger		0.7		.02
Avoidance Focused Coping Strategies		.23**		.08
Step 2	.00		.00	
State Anger				-.06
* Avoidance Focused Coping Strategies		-.04		
R^2	.03**		.07	

**** $p < .01$, * $p < .05$.**

Table 67 illustrates moderation analysis for avoidance focused coping strategies in the relationship between State Anger and Psychological well-being (environmental mastery and personal growth). Avoidance focused coping strategies are not acting as a moderator for the relationship of state anger with environmental mastery and personal growth.

Table 68

Moderating Effect of Religious focused coping strategies on Relationship of State Anger with Environmental Mastery and Personal Growth (n = 500)

Variables	Environmental Mastery		Personal growth	
	$\triangle R^2$	β	$\triangle R^2$	β
Step 1				
State Anger		.11*		.07
Religious Focused Coping Strategies		-.07		-.13**
Step 2	.00		.01	
State Anger				-.13
* Religious Focused Coping Strategies		-.10		
R^2	.01		.02*	

*** $p < .01$, * $p < .05$.*

Table 68 illustrates moderation analysis for religious focused coping strategies in the relationship between State Anger and Psychological well-being (environmental mastery and personal growth). Religious focused coping strategies are not acting as a moderator for the relationship of state anger with environmental mastery and personal growth.

Table 69

Moderating Effect of Active distracting coping strategies on Relationship of State Anger with Environmental Mastery and Personal Growth (n = 500)

Variables	Environmental Mastery		Personal growth	
	$\triangle R^2$	β	$\triangle R^2$	β
Step 1				
State Anger		.01		-.02
Active Distracting Coping Strategies		.04		-.02
Step 2	.04***		.02**	
State Anger				-.12**
* Active Distracting Coping Strategies		-.18***		
R^2	.04***		.14**	

*** p < .01, * p < .05.*

Table 69 illustrates moderation analysis for active distracting coping strategies in the relationship between State Anger and Psychological well-being (environmental mastery and personal growth). Active distracting coping strategies are acting as a moderator for the relationship of state anger with environmental mastery and personal growth. This added additional 4% of the variance is explained by the relationship (environmental mastery and state anger) which is moderated by active focused coping strategies. The additional 2% of the variance is explained by the relationship (personal growth and state anger) which is moderated by the active focused coping strategies. The moderating effect is further explained through mod graphs.

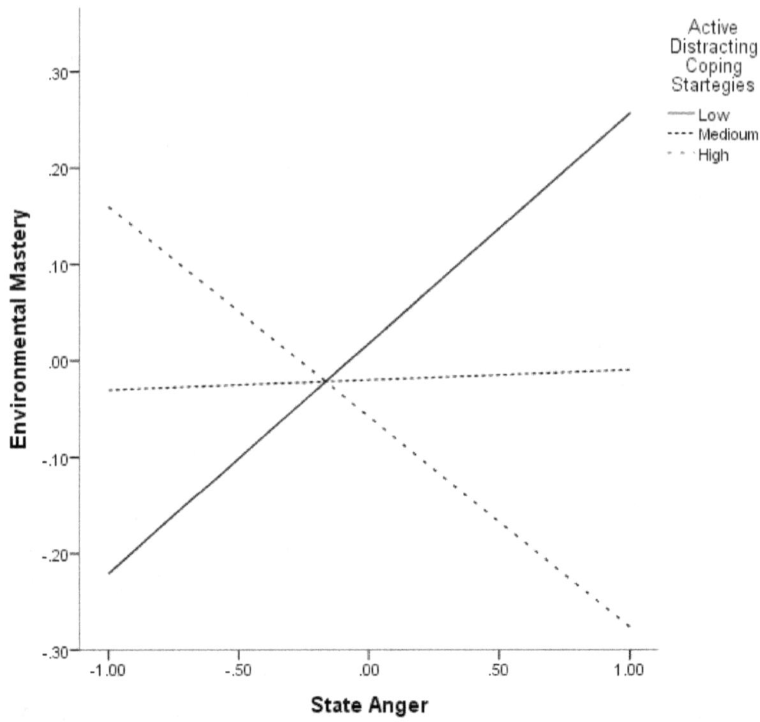

Figure 45. Active distracting coping strategies as a moderator between environmental mastery and state anger

The correlation of state anger with environmental mastery is moderated by the Active distracting coping strategies. When the Active distracting coping strategies is increasingly used by the patients, the relationship between state anger and environmental mastery is negative, which means that in case if the patients are using the Active distracting coping strategies the state anger increases and environmental mastery decreases.

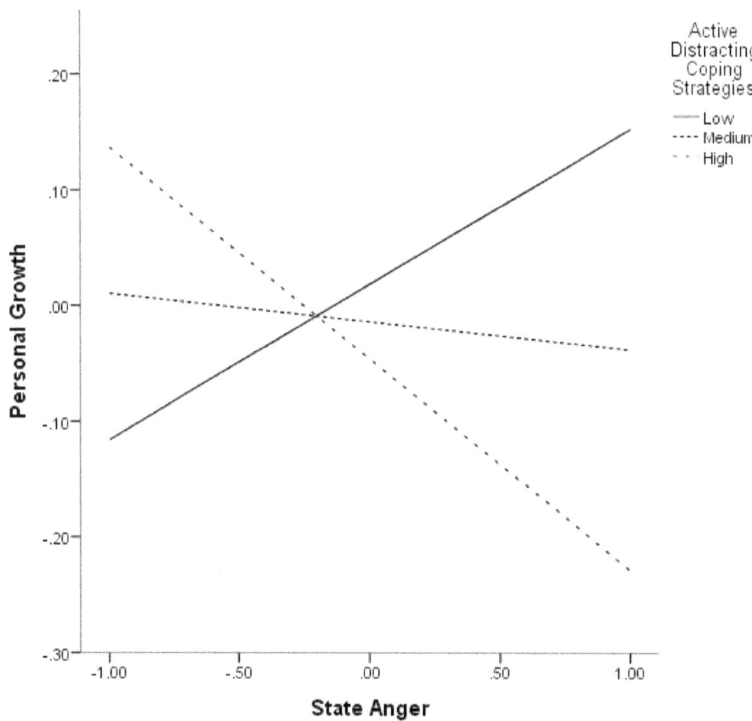

Figure 46. Active distracting coping strategies as a moderator between personal growth and state anger

The correlation of state anger with personal growth is moderated by the Active distracting coping strategies. When the Active distracting coping strategies is increasingly used by the patients, the relationship between state anger and personal growth is negative, which means that in case if the patients are using the Active distracting coping strategies the state anger increases and personal growth decreases.

Table 70

Moderating Effect of Informational Support on Relationship of State Anger with Environmental Mastery and Personal Growth (n = 500)

Variables	Environmental Mastery		Personal growth	
	ΔR^2	β	ΔR^2	β
Step 1				
State Anger		-.07		-.09
Informational support		-.29***		-.28***
Step 2	.03***		.01*	
State Anger		-.16***		-.11*
* Informational support				
R^2	.12***		.31***	

** $p < .01$, * $p < .05$.

Table 70 illustrates moderation analysis for informational support in the relationship between State Anger and Psychological well-being (environmental mastery and personal growth). Informational support is acting as a moderator for the relationship of state anger with environmental mastery and personal growth. This added additional 3% of the variance is explained by the relationship (environmental mastery and state anger) which is moderated by informational support. The additional 1% of the variance is explained by the relationship (personal growth and state anger) which is moderated by the informational support. The moderating effect is further explained through mod graphs.

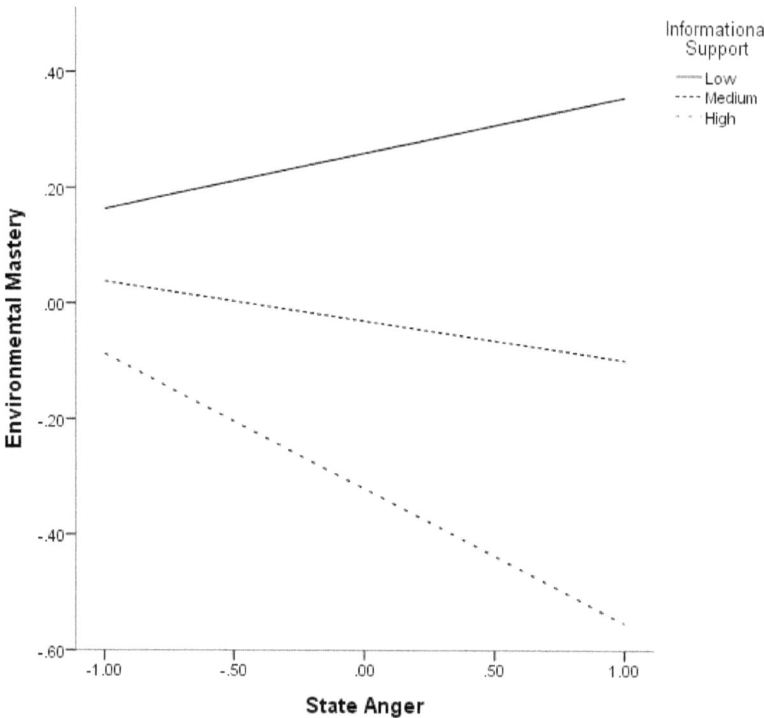

Figure 47. Informational support as a moderator between environmental mastery and state anger

The correlation between the state anger with environmental mastery is moderated by the Informational support. When the informational support is increasingly used by the patients, the relationship between state anger and environmental mastery is negative, which means that in case if the patients are using the informational support the state anger increases and environmental mastery decreases.

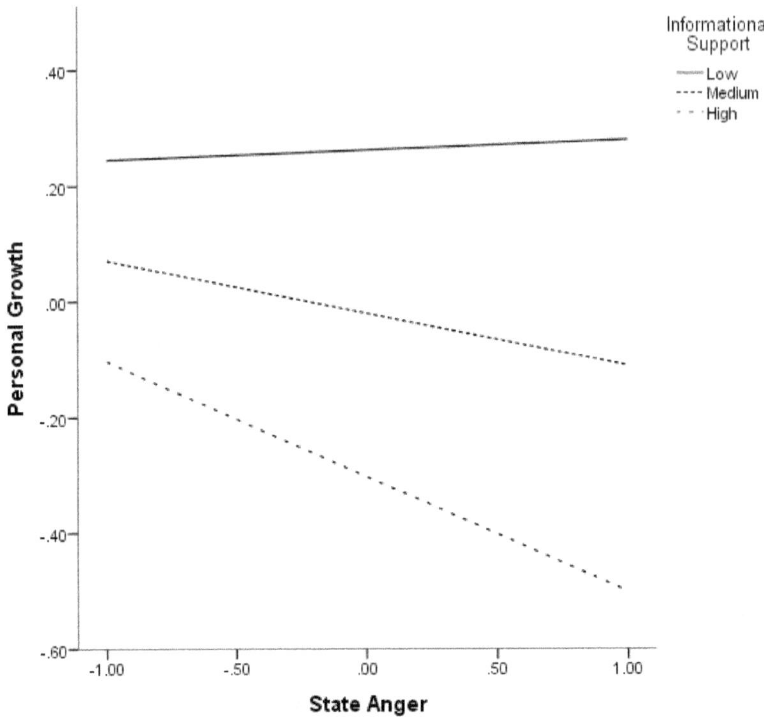

Figure 48. Informational support as a moderator between personal growth and state anger

The correlation of state anger with personal growth is moderated by the Informational support. When the informational support is increasingly used by the patients, the relationship between state anger and personal growth is negative, which means that in case if the patients are using the informational support the state anger increases and personal growth decreases.

Table 71

Moderating Effect of Tangible Support on Relationship of State Anger with Environmental Mastery and Personal Growth (n = 500)

Variables	Environmental Mastery		Personal growth	
	$\triangle R^2$	β	$\triangle R^2$	β
Step 1				
State Anger		-.18**		-.19**
Tangible support		-.29***		-.30***
Step 2	.042***		.02**	
State Anger * Tangible support		-.18***		-.13**
R^2	.37***		.12***	

*** p < .01, * p < .05.*

Table 71 illustrates moderation analysis for informational support in the relationship between State Anger and Psychological well-being (environmental mastery and personal growth). Informational support is acting as a moderator for the relationship of state anger with environmental mastery and personal growth. This added additional 3% of the variance is explained by the relationship (environmental mastery and state anger) which is moderated by informational support. The additional 1% of the variance is explained by the relationship (personal growth and state anger) which is moderated by the informational support. The moderating effect is further explained through mod graphs.

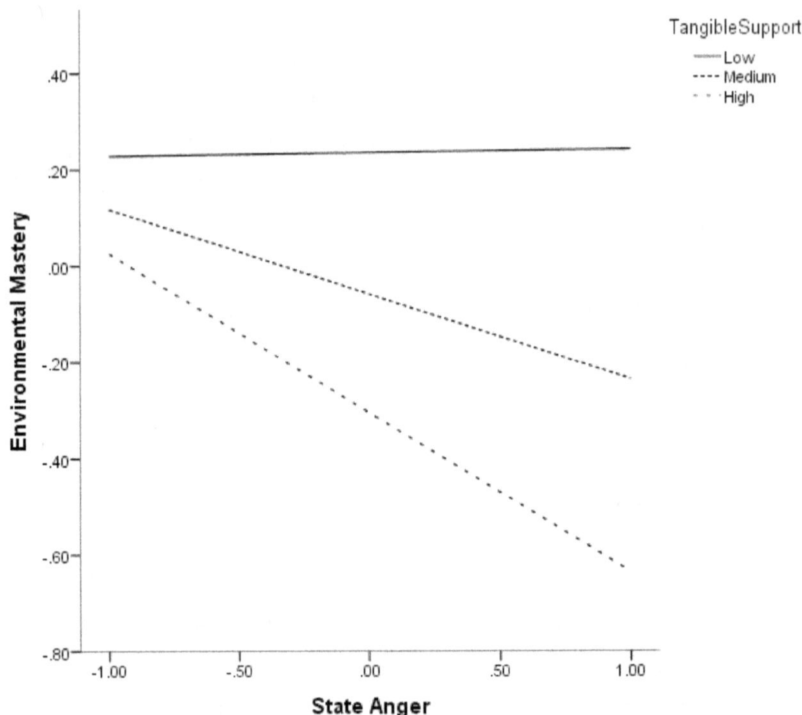

Figure 49. Tangible support as a moderator between environmental mastery and state anger

The correlation of state anger with environmental mastery is moderated by the tangible support. When the tangible support is increasingly used by the patients, the relationship between state anger and environmental mastery is negative, which means that in case if the patients are using the tangible support the state anger increases and environmental mastery decreases.

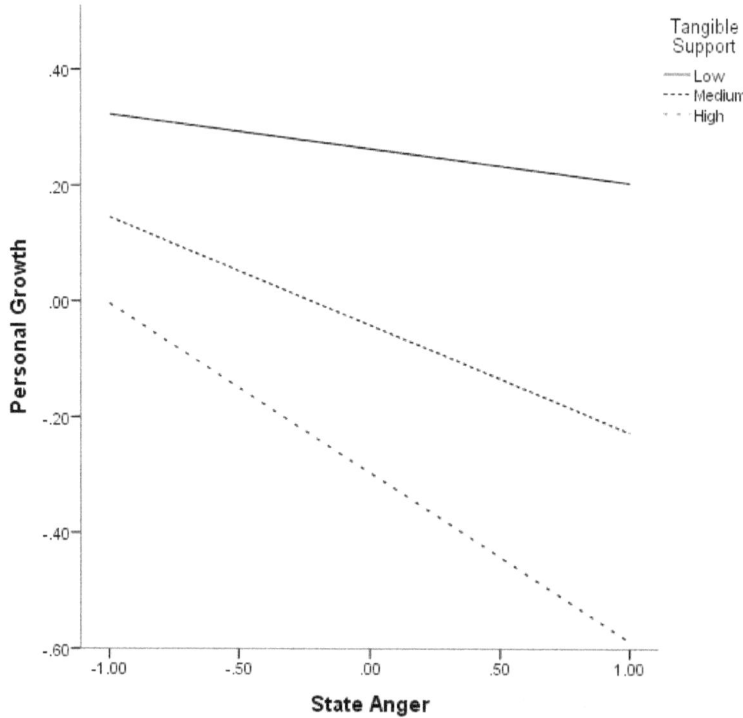

Figure 50. Tangible support as a moderator between personal growth and state anger

The correlation of state anger with personal growth is moderated by the tangible support. When the tangible support is increasingly used by the patients, the relationship between state anger and personal growth is negative, which means that in case if the patients are using the tangible support the state anger increases and personal growth decreases.

Table 72

Moderating Effect of Emotional Support on Relationship of State Anger with Environmental Mastery and Personal Growth (n = 500)

Variables	Environmental Mastery		Personal growth	
	$\triangle R^2$	β	$\triangle R^2$	β
Step 1				
State Anger		-.21**		-.20**
Emotional support		.36		-.06
Step 2	.06***		.03**	
State Anger				-.13**
* Emotional support		-.18***		
R^2	.09***		.05***	

** $p < .01$, * $p < .05$.

Table 72 illustrates moderation analysis for emotional support in the relationship between State Anger and Psychological well-being (environmental mastery and personal growth). Emotional support is acting as a moderator for the relationship of state anger with environmental mastery and personal growth. This added additional 6% of the variance is explained by the relationship (environmental mastery and state anger) which is moderated by emotional support. The additional 3% of the variance is explained by the relationship (personal growth and state anger) which is moderated by the emotional support. The moderating effect is further explained through mod graphs.

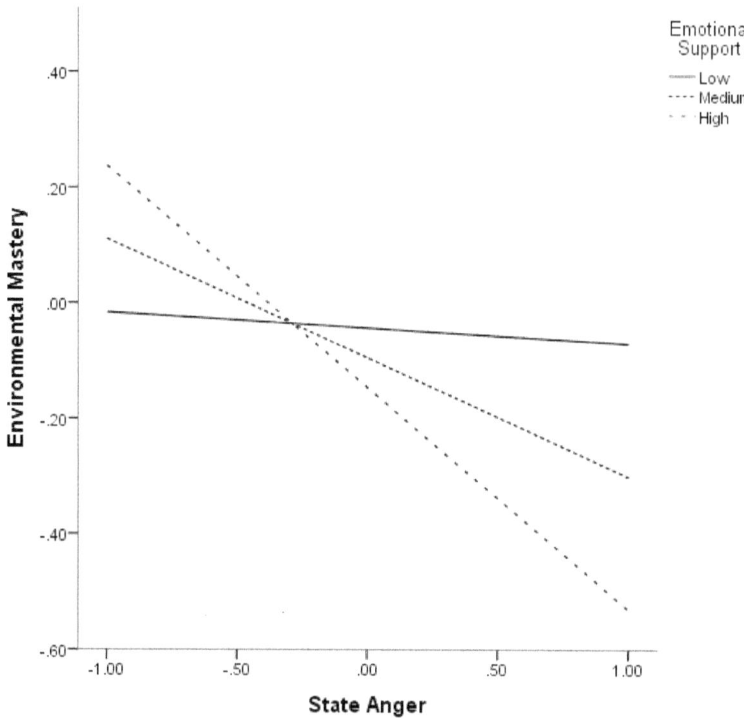

Figure 51. Emotional Support as a moderator between environmental mastery and state anger

The correlation of state anger with environmental mastery is moderated by the emotional support. When the emotional support is increasingly used by the patients, the relationship between state anger and environmental mastery is negative, which means that in case if the patients are using the emotional support the state anger increases and environmental mastery decreases.

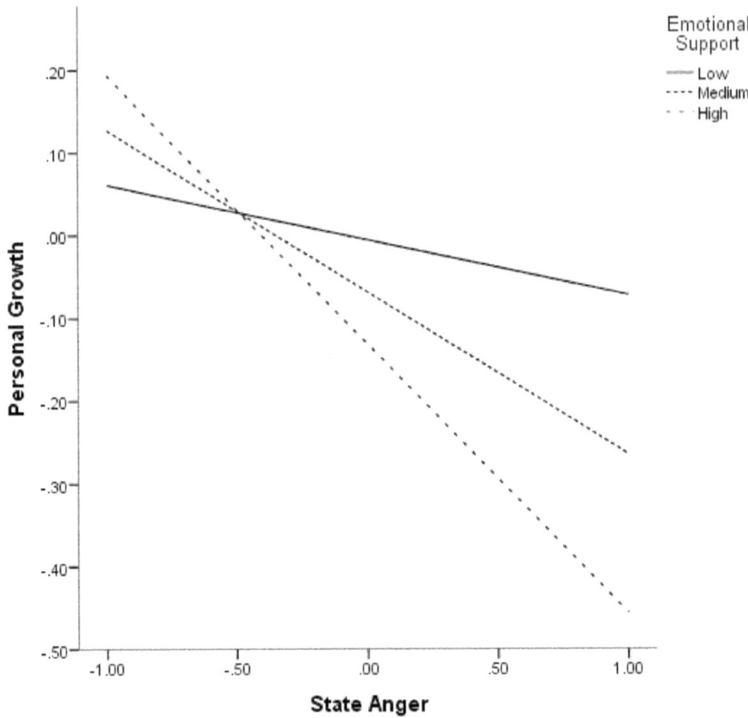

Figure 52. Emotional Support as a moderator between personal growth and state anger

The correlation between the state anger with personal growth is moderated by the emotional support. When the emotional support is increasingly used by the patients, the relationship between state anger and personal growth is negative, which means that in case if the patients are using the emotional support the state anger increases and personal growth decreases.

Table 73

Moderating Effect of Self-Esteem Support on Relationship of State Anger with Environmental Mastery and Personal Growth (n = 500)

Variables	Environmental Mastery		Personal growth	
	$\triangle R^2$	β	$\triangle R^2$	β
Step 1				
State Anger		-.27***		-.26***
Self-Esteem support		-.13*		-.21**
Step 2	-.06***		.02**	
State Anger * Self-Esteem support		-.20***		-.12**
R^2	.11***		.08***	

$** p < .01, * p < .05.$

Table 73 illustrates moderation analysis for self-esteem support in the relationship between State Anger and Psychological well-being (environmental mastery and personal growth). Self-esteem is acting as a moderator for the relationship of state anger with environmental mastery and personal growth. This added additional 6% of the variance is explained by the relationship (environmental mastery and state anger) which is moderated by self-esteem support. The additional 2% of the variance is explained by the relationship (personal growth and state anger) which is moderated by the self-esteem support. The moderating effect is further explained through mod graphs.

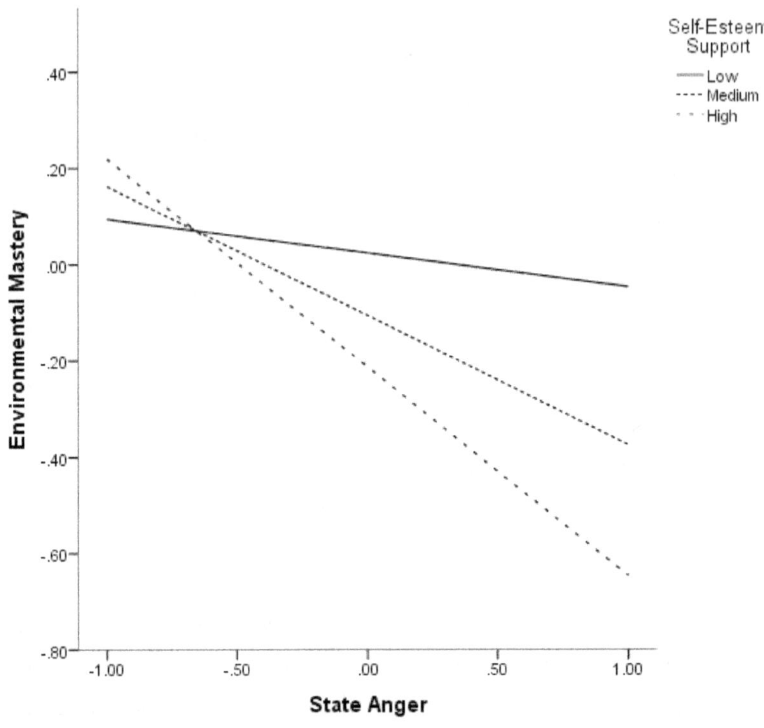

Figure 53. Self-Esteem Support as a moderator between environmental mastery and state anger

The correlation of state anger with environmental mastery is moderated by the self-esteem support. When the self-esteem support is increasingly used by the patients, the relationship between state anger and environmental mastery is negative, which means that in case if the patients are using the self-esteem support the state anger increases and environmental mastery decreases.

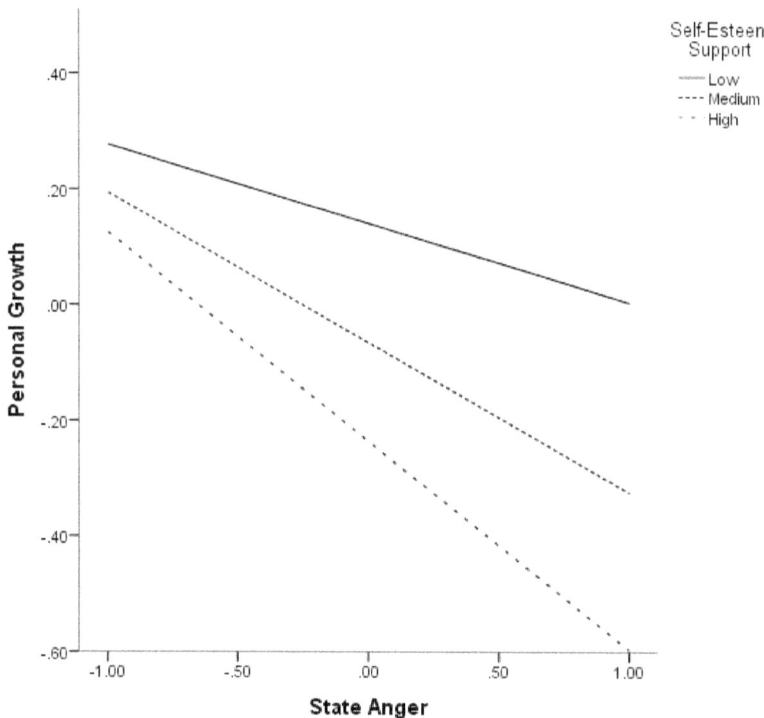

Figure 54. Self-Esteem Support as a moderator between personal growth and state anger

The correlation of state anger with personal growth is moderated by the self-esteem support. When the self-esteem support is increasingly used by the patients, the relationship between state anger and personal growth is negative, which means that in case if the patients are using the self-esteem support the state anger increases and personal growth decreases.

Table 74

Moderating Effect of Social networking Support on Relationship of State Anger with Environmental Mastery and Personal Growth (n = 500)

Variables	Environmental Mastery		Personal growth	
	$\triangle R^2$	β	$\triangle R^2$	β
Step 1				
State Anger		-.14*		-.14**
Social networking support		-.12**		-.22***
Step 2	.06***		.02**	
State Anger * Social networking support		-.24***		-.13**
R^2	.27***		.06***	

** $p < .01$, * $p < .05$.

Table 74 illustrates moderation analysis for social networking support in the relationship between State Anger and Psychological well-being (environmental mastery and personal growth). Social networking is acting as a moderator for the relationship of state anger with environmental mastery and personal growth. This added additional 6% of the variance is explained by the relationship (environmental mastery and state anger) which is moderated by social networking support. The additional 2% of the variance is explained by the relationship (personal growth and state anger) which is moderated by the social networking support. The moderating effect is further explained through mod graphs.

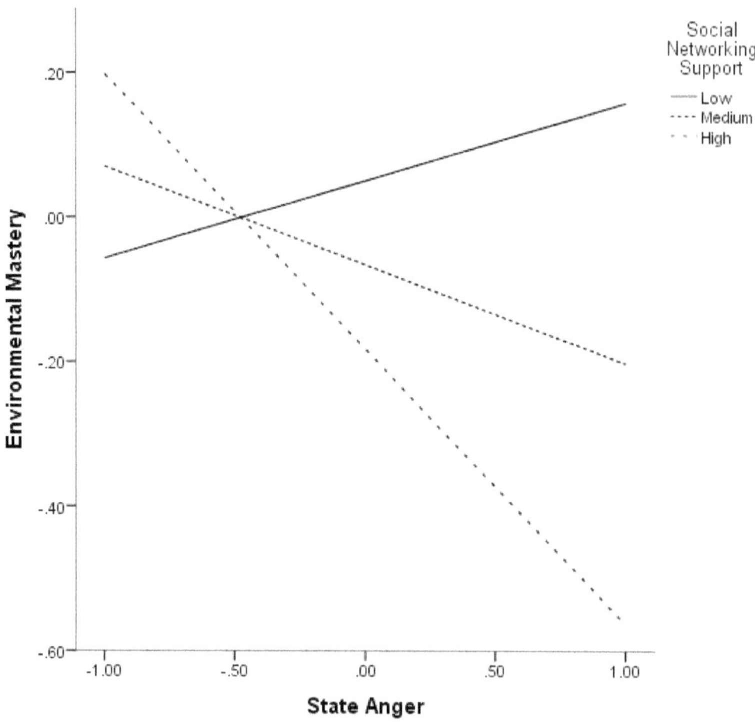

Figure 55. Social networking Support as a moderator between environmental mastery and state anger

The correlation of state anger with environmental mastery is moderated by the social networking support. When the social networking support is increasingly used by the patients, the relationship between state anger and environmental mastery is negative, which means that in case if the patients are using the social networking support the state anger increases and environmental mastery decreases.

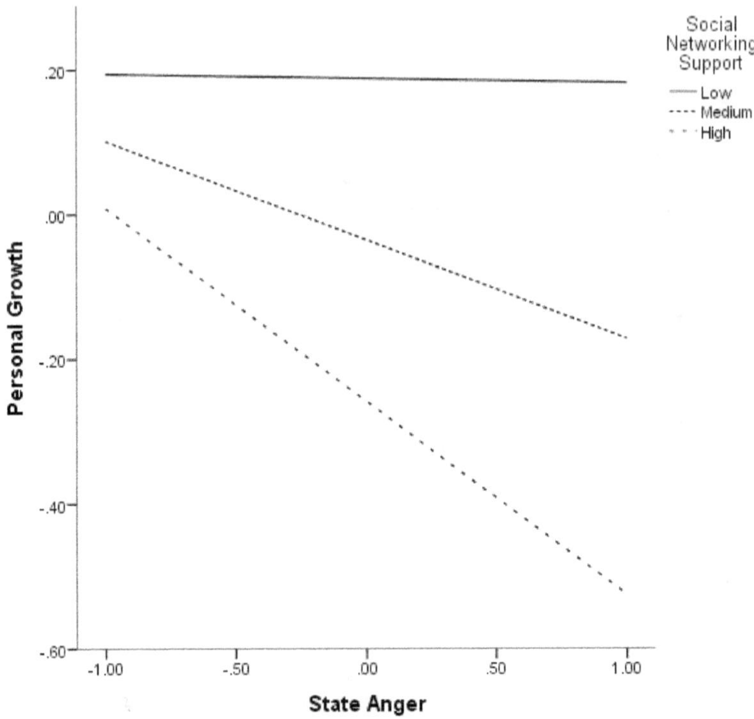

Figure 56. Self-Esteem Support as a moderator between personal growth and state anger

The correlation between the state anger with personal growth is moderated by the social networking support. When the social networking support is increasingly used by the patients, the relationship between state anger and personal growth is negative, which means that in case if the patients are using the social networking support the state anger increases and personal growth decreases.

Table 75

Moderating Effect of Active Focused Coping Strategies on Relationship of State Anger with Psychological Functioning, Social Relationships and Environment (n = 500)

Variables	Psychological Functioning		Social Relationships		Environment	
	ΔR^2	β	ΔR^2	β	ΔR^2	β
Step 1						
State Anger		-.42		2.26*		2.87*
Active focused coping strategies		5.38***		9.88***		19.91***
Step 2	.00		.00		.00	
State Anger				.25		-.05
* Active focused coping strategies		-.04				
R^2	.13***		.35***		.41***	

*** p < .01, * p < .05.*

Table 75 illustrates moderation analysis for active focused coping strategies in the relationship between State Anger and Quality of life (psychological functioning, social relationships and environment). Active focused coping strategies are acting as a moderator for the relationship of state anger with psychological functioning, social relationships and environment.

Table 76

Moderating Effect of Avoidance focused coping strategies on Relationship of State Anger with Psychological functioning, Social relationships and Environment (n = 500)

Variables	Psychological Functioning		Social Relationships		Environment	
	ΔR^2	β	ΔR^2	β	ΔR^2	β
Step 1						
State Anger		-3.07***		6.96***		-7.58***
Avoidance focused coping strategies		7.44***		-3.09***		23.67***
Step 2	.00		.00		.00	
State Anger						2.58
* Avoidance focused coping strategies		-.88		.95		
R^2		.16***		.13***		.35***

** $p < .01$, * $p < .05$.

Table 76 illustrates moderation analysis for avoidance focused coping strategies in the relationship between State Anger and Quality of life (psychological functioning, social relationships and environment). Avoidance focused coping strategies are acting as a moderator for the relationship of state anger with psychological functioning, social relationships and environment.

Table 77

Moderating Effect of Religious focused coping strategies on Relationship of State Anger with Psychological Functioning, Social Relationships and Environment (n = 500)

Variables	Psychological Functioning		Social Relationships		Environment	
	ΔR^2	β	ΔR^2	β	ΔR^2	β
Step 1						
State Anger		-3.26***		-3.92***		-9.37***
Religious focused coping strategies		1.97**		5.57***		14.54***
Step 2	.00		.00		.01**	
State Anger				1.60		3.55**
* Religious focused coping strategies		.26				
R^2	.06***		.21***		.63***	

** $p < .01$, * $p < .05$.

Table 77 illustrates moderation analysis for religious focused coping strategies in the relationship between State Anger and Quality of life (psychological functioning, social relationships and environment). Religious focused coping strategies are acting as a moderator for the relationship of state anger with environment. This added additional 1% of the variance is explained by the relationship between state anger and environment which is moderated by religious focused coping strategies. The moderating effect is further explained through mod graphs.

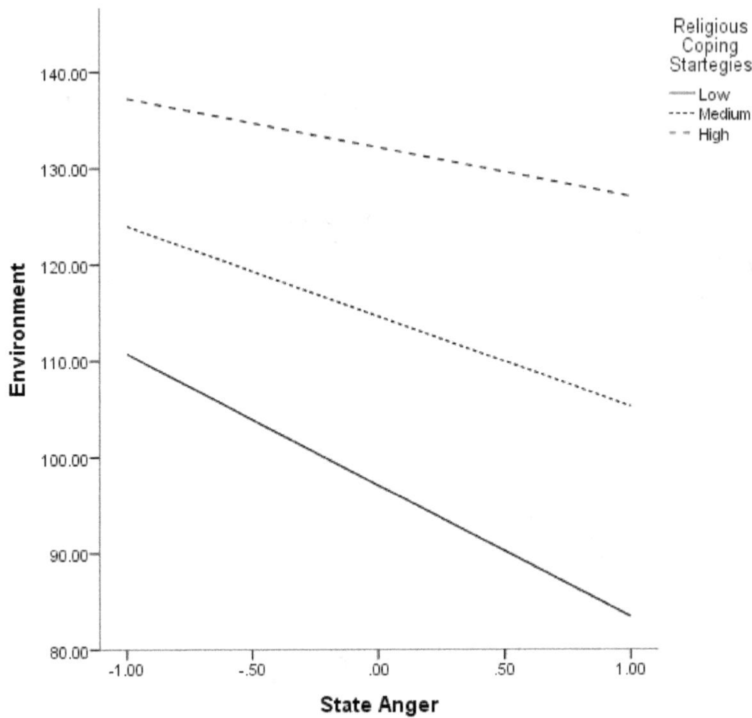

Figure 57. Religious focused coping strategies as a moderator between environment and state anger

The correlation of state anger with environment is moderated by the religious focused coping strategies. When the religious focused coping strategies are increasingly used by the patients, the relationship between state anger and environment is negative, which means that in case if the patients are using the religious focused coping strategies the state anger increases and environment decreases.

Table 78

Moderating Effect of Active distracting coping strategies on Relationship of State Anger with Psychological functioning, Social relationships and Environment (n = 500)

Variables	Psychological Functioning		Social Relationships		Environment	
	$\triangle R^2$	β	$\triangle R^2$	β	$\triangle R^2$	β
Step 1						
State Anger		-2.40**		-1.78**		-3.67**
Active distracting coping strategies		2.03**		2.61***		12.86***
Step 2	.01		.03**		.02***	
State Anger				2.21**		3.67***
* Active distracting coping strategies		1.01				
R^2	.07***		.11***		.40***	

** $p < .01$, * $p < .05$.

Table 78 illustrates moderation analysis for active distracting coping strategies in the relationship between State Anger and Quality of life (psychological functioning, social relationships and environment). Active distracting coping strategies are acting as a moderator for the relationship of state anger with social relationships and environment. This added additional 3% of the variance is explained by the relationship between state anger and social relationships which is moderated by active distracting coping strategies. This added additional 2% of the variance is explained by the relationship between state anger and environment which is moderated by active distracting coping strategies. The moderating effect is further explained through mod graphs.

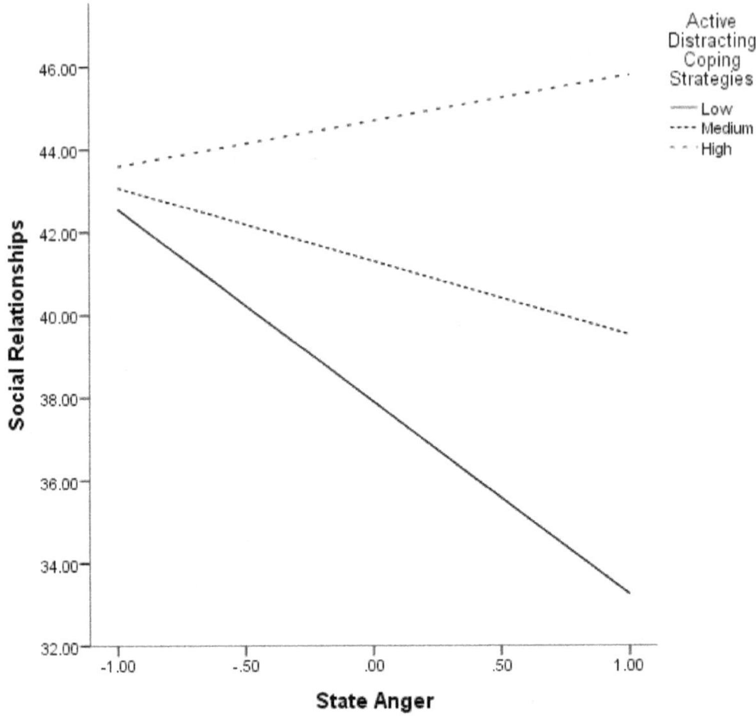

Figure 58. Active distracting coping strategies as a moderator between social relationships and state anger

The correlation between the state anger with social relationships is moderated by the active distracting coping strategies. When the active distracting coping strategies are increasingly used by the patients, the relationship between state anger and social relationships is negative, which means that in case if the patients are using the active distracting coping strategies the state anger increases and social relationships decreases.

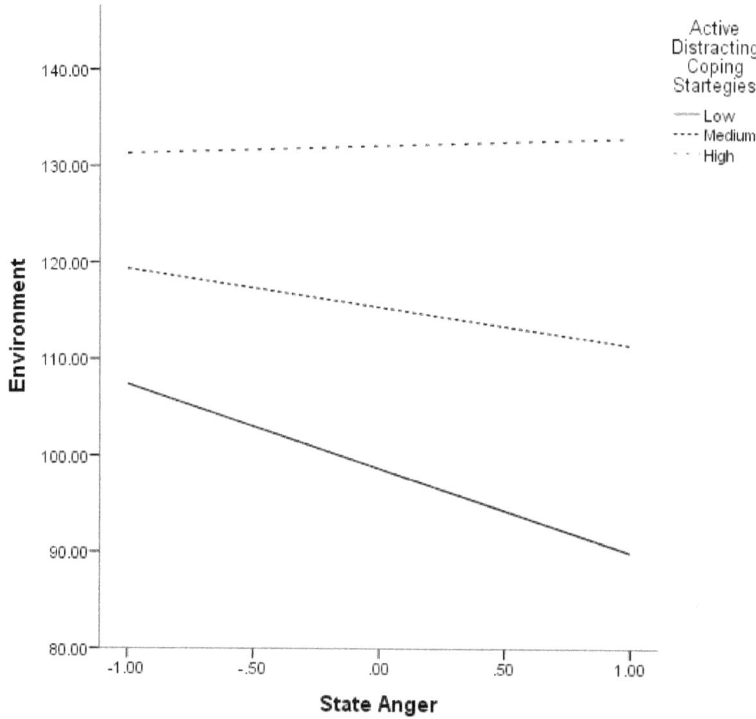

Figure 59. Active distracting coping strategies as a moderator between environment and state anger

The correlation of state anger with environment is moderated by the active distracting coping strategies. When the active distracting coping strategies are increasingly used by the patients, the relationship between state anger and environment is negative, which means that in case if the patients are using the active distracting coping strategies the state anger increases and environment decreases.

Table 79

Moderating Effect of Informational Support on Relationship of State Anger with Psychological Functioning, Social Relationships and Environment (n = 500)

Variables	Psychological Functioning		Social Relationships		Environment	
	ΔR^2	β	ΔR^2	β	ΔR^2	β
Step 1						
State Anger		-1.78**		-1.02		-2.55*
Informational Support		1.25		4.25***		10.73**
Step 2	.02**		.02*		.02**	
State Anger * Informational support		1.85**		1.89*		3.10**
R^2	.06***		.13***		.22***	

** $p < .01$, * $p < .05$.

Table 79 illustrates moderation analysis for informational support in the relationship between State Anger and Quality of life (psychological functioning, social relationships and environment). Informational support is acting as a moderator for the relationship of state anger with psychological functioning, social relationships and environment. This added additional 2% of the variance is explained by the relationship between state anger and psychological functioning which is moderated by Informational support. This added additional 2% of the variance is explained by the relationship between state anger and social relationships which is moderated by Informational support. This added additional 2% of the variance is explained by the relationship between state anger and environment which is moderated by Informational support. The moderating effect is further explained through mod graphs.

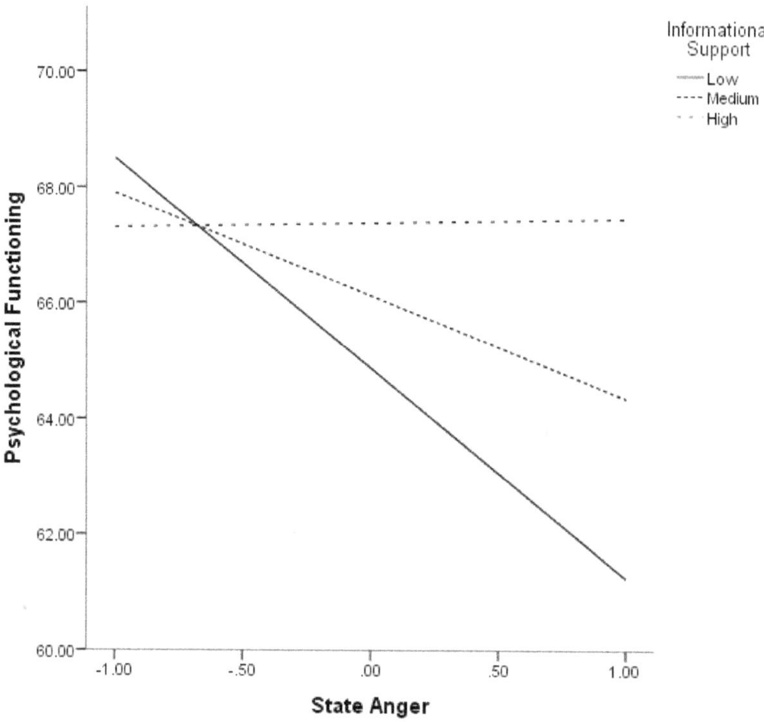

Figure 60. Informational Support as a moderator between psychological functioning and state anger

The correlation between the state anger with psychological functioning is moderated by the informational support. When the informational support is increasingly used by the patients, the relationship between state anger and psychological functioning is negative, which means that in case if the patients are using the informational support the state anger increases and psychological functioning decreases.

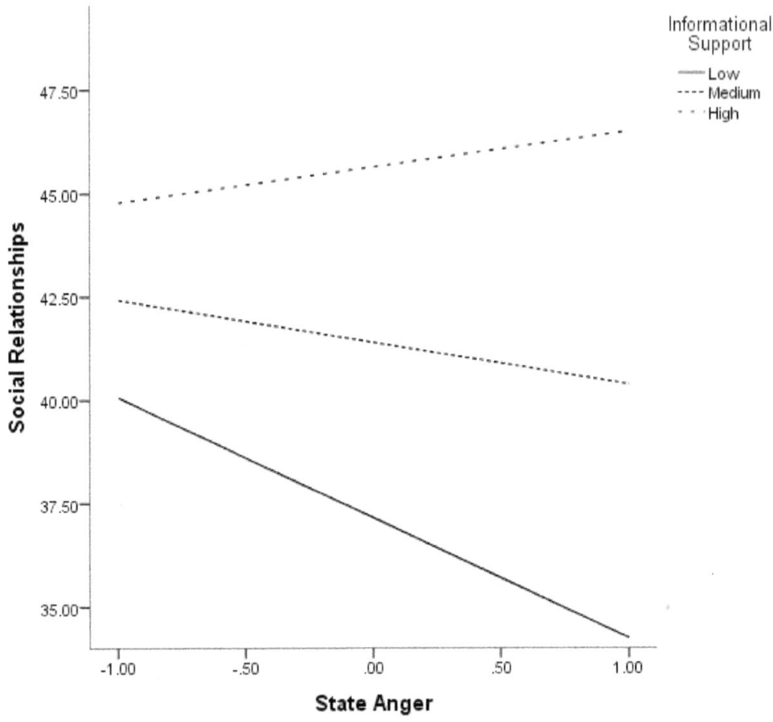

Figure 61. Informational Support as a moderator between social relationships and state anger

The correlation of state anger with social relationships is moderated by the informational support. When the informational support is increasingly used by the patients, the relationship between state anger and social relationships is negative, which means that in case if the patients are using the informational support the state anger increases and social relationships decreases.

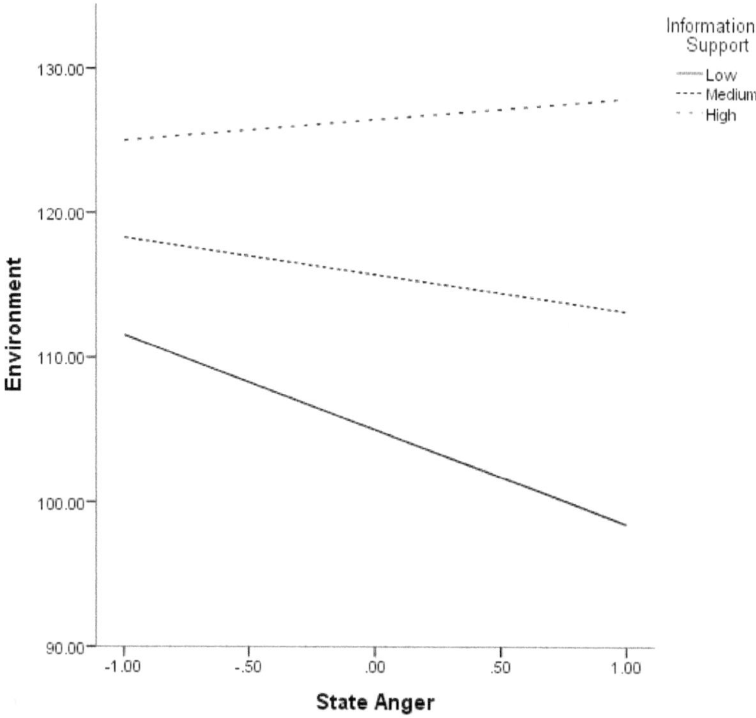

Figure 62. Informational Support as a moderator between environment and state anger

The correlation of state anger with environment is moderated by the informational support. When the informational support is increasingly used by the patients, the relationship between state anger and environment is negative, which means that in case if the patients are using the informational support the state anger increases and environment decreases.

Table 80

Moderating Effect of Tangible Support on Relationship of State Anger with Psychological Functioning, Social Relationships and Environment (n = 500)

Variables	Psychological Functioning		Social Relationships		Environment	
	ΔR^2	β	ΔR^2	β	ΔR^2	β
Step 1						
State Anger		-.69		.39		-.11
Tangible Support		4.18***		5.15***		12.97***
Step 2	.01*		.02**		.012*	
State Anger * Tangible support		1.10*		1.82**		2.76*
R^2	.12***		.17***		.27***	

** $p < .01$, * $p < .05$.

Table 80 illustrates moderation analysis for tangible support in the relationship between State Anger and Quality of life (psychological functioning, social relationships and environment). Tangible support is acting as a moderator for the relationship of state anger with psychological functioning, social relationships and environment. This added additional 1% of the variance is explained by the relationship between state anger and psychological functioning which is moderated by tangible support. This added additional 2% of the variance is explained by the relationship between state anger and social relationships which is moderated by tangible support. This added additional 1.2% of the variance is explained by the relationship between state anger and environment which is moderated by tangible support. The moderating effect is further explained through mod graphs.

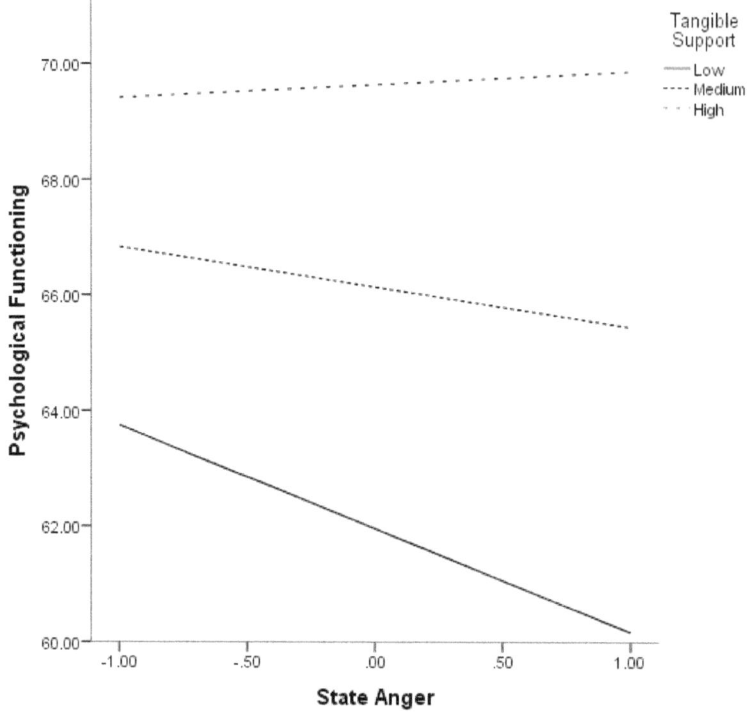

Figure 63. Tangible Support as a moderator between psychological functioning and state anger

The correlation of state anger with psychological functioning is moderated by the tangible support. When the tangible support is increasingly used by the patients, the relationship between state anger and psychological functioning is negative, which means that in case if the patients are using the tangible support the state anger increases and psychological functioning decreases.

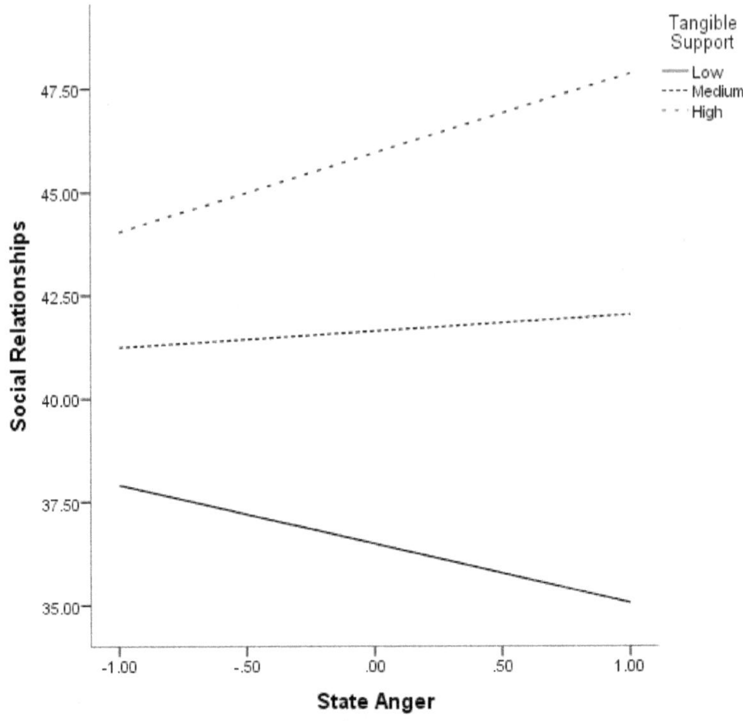

Figure 64. Tangible Support as a moderator between social relationships and state anger

The correlation of state anger with social relationships is moderated by the tangible support. When the tangible support is increasingly used by the patients, the relationship between state anger and social relationships is positive, which means that in case if the patients are using the tangible support the state anger increases and social relationships increase.

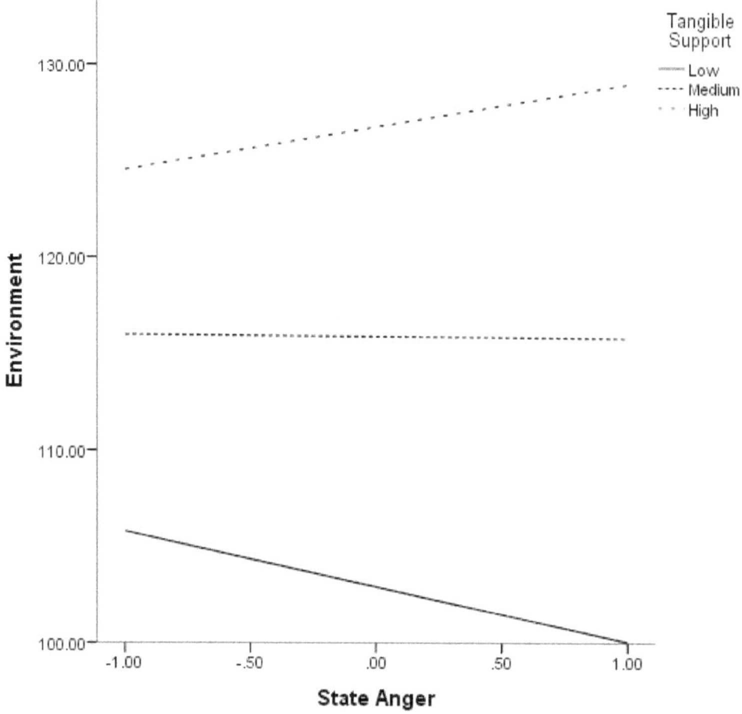

Figure 65. Tangible Support as a moderator between environment and state anger

The correlation of state anger with environment is moderated by the tangible support. When the tangible support is increasingly used by the patients, the relationship between state anger and environment is negative, which means that in case if the patients are using the tangible support the state anger increases and environment decreases. But as according to scoring if the scores are low in support it indicates that the support is high and if scored are high the support is low. So if the person is having less tangible support the relationship between the state anger and environment is negative and state anger is high and environment are low.

Table 81

Moderating Effect of Self-Esteem Support on Relationship of State Anger with Psychological Functioning, Social Relationships and Environment (n = 500)

Variables	Psychological Functioning		Social Relationships		Environment	
	ΔR^2	β	ΔR^2	β	ΔR^2	β
Step 1						
State Anger		-.21		2.34*		4.15*
Self-Esteem Support		5.59***		8.52***		21.88***
Step 2	.00		.00		.00	
State Anger				.40		-.74
* Self-Esteem support		-.19				
R^2	.14***		.28***		.47***	

$**\,p < .01, *\,p < .05.$

Table 81 illustrates moderation analysis for esteem support in the relationship between State Anger and Quality of life (psychological functioning, social relationships and environment). Esteem support is not acting as a moderator for the relationship of state anger with psychological functioning, social relationships and environment.

Table 82

Moderating Effect of Emotional Support on Relationship of State Anger with Psychological Functioning, Social Relationships and Environment (n = 500)

Variables	Psychological Functioning		Social Relationships		Environment	
	$\triangle R^2$	β	$\triangle R^2$	β	$\triangle R^2$	β
Step 1						
State Anger		-.37		1.48		2.87*
Emotional Support		6.73***		6.77***		24.63***
Step 2	.00		.00		.02**	
State Anger				.48		-2.65**
* Emotional Support		-.72				
R^2	.17***		.20***		.53***	

**$p < .01$, *$p < .05$.

Table 82 illustrates moderation analysis for emotional support in the relationship between State Anger and Quality of life (psychological functioning, social relationships and environment). Emotional support is acting as a moderator for the relationship of state anger with environment. This added additional 2% of the variance is explained by the relationship between state anger and environment which is moderated by tangible support. The moderating effect is further explained through mod graphs.

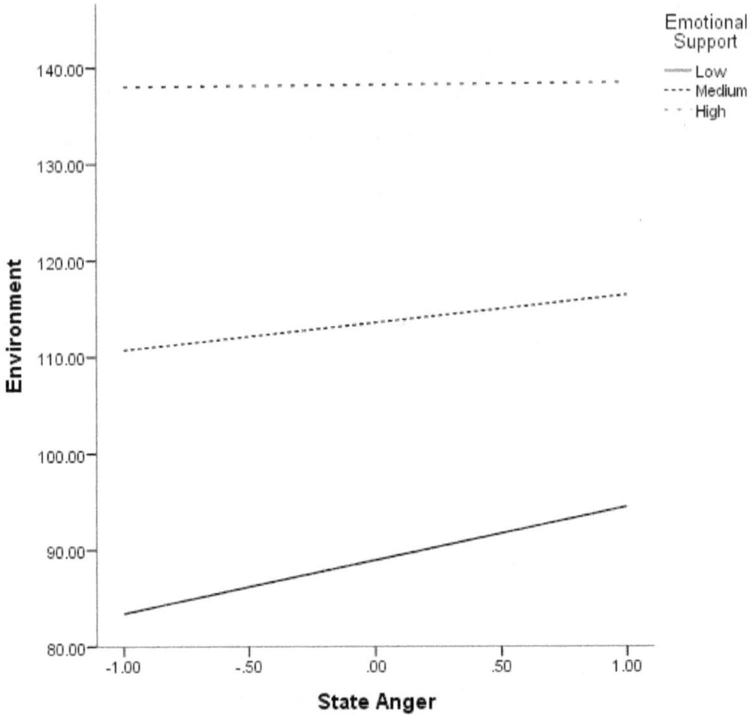

Figure 66. Emotional Support as a moderator between environment and state anger

The correlation of state anger with environment is moderated by the emotional support. When the emotional support is increasingly used by the patients, the relationship between state anger and environment is negative, which means that in case if the patients are using the emotional support the state anger increases and environment decreases. But as according to scoring if the scores are low in support it indicates that the support is high and if scored are high the support is low. So if the person is having less emotional support the relationship between the state anger and environment is negative and state anger is high and environment are low.

Table 83

Moderating Effect of Social Networking Support on Relationship of State Anger with Psychological Functioning, Social Relationships and Environment (n = 500)

Variables	Psychological Functioning		Social Relationships		Environment	
	$\triangle R^2$	β	$\triangle R^2$	β	$\triangle R^2$	β
Step 1						
State Anger		-.84		.89		1.14
Social Networking Support		8.75***		8.70***		23.50***
Step 2	.00		.01**		.00**	
State Anger * Social Networking Support		-.37		1.83**		1.90**
R^2	.36***		.36***		.70***	

*** p < .01, * p < .05.*

Table 83 illustrates moderation analysis for social networking support in the relationship between State Anger and Quality of life (psychological functioning, social relationships and environment). Social Networking Support is acting as a moderator for the relationship of state anger with environment. This added additional 1% of the variance is explained by the relationship between state anger and social networking which is moderated by social networking support. This added additional 0% of the variance is explained by the relationship between state anger and environment which is moderated by social networking support. The moderating effect is further explained through mod graphs.

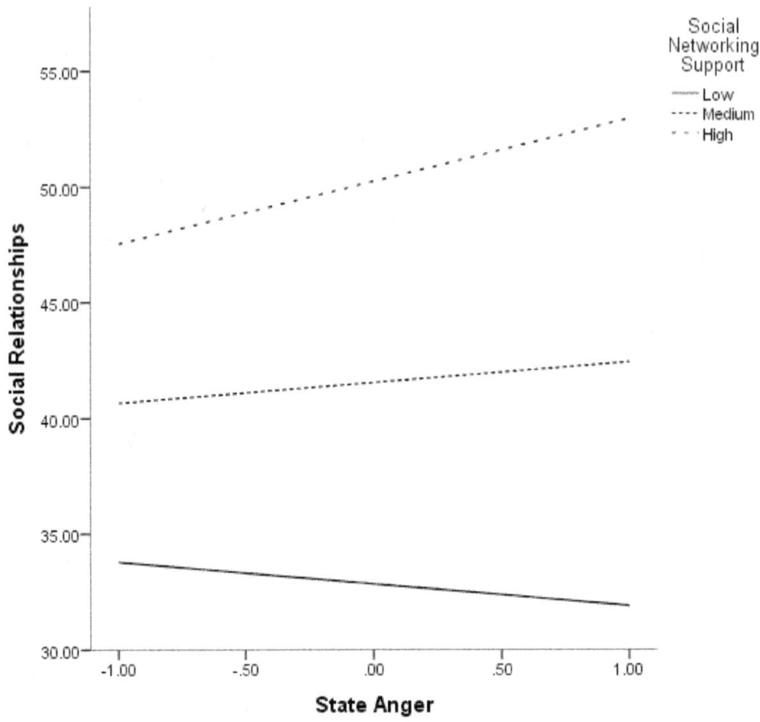

Figure 67. Social Networking Support as a moderator between environment and state anger

The correlation between the state anger with social relationships is moderated by the social networking support. When the social networking support is increasingly used by the patients, the relationship between state anger and social relationships is negative, which means that in case if the patients are using the social networking support the state anger increases and social relationships decreases. But as according to scoring if the scores are low in support it indicates that the support is high and if scored are high the support is low. So if the person is having less social networking support the relationship between the state anger and social relationships is negative and state anger is high and social relationships are low.

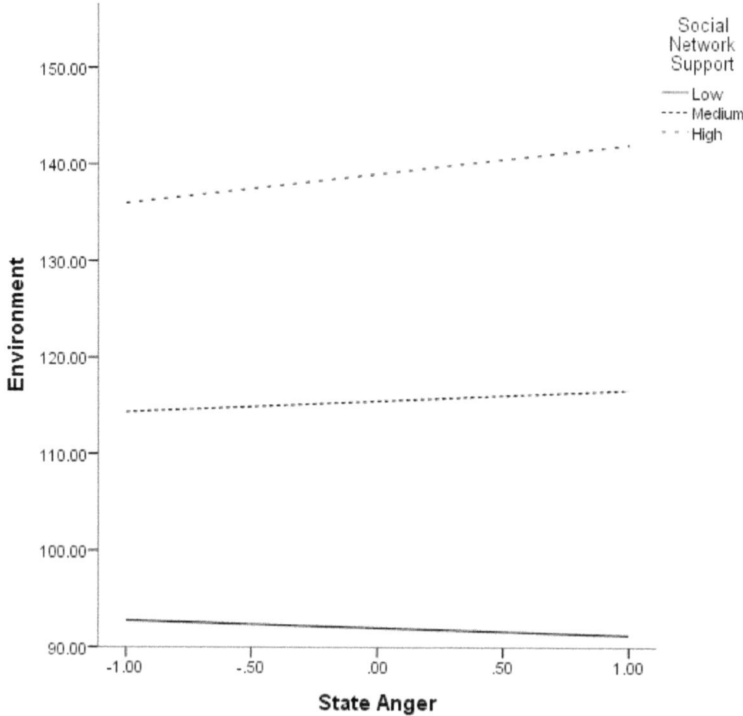

Figure 68. Social Networking Support as a moderator between environment and state anger

The correlation between the state anger with environment is moderated by the social networking support. When the social networking support is increasingly used by the patients, the relationship between state anger and environment is negative, which means that in case if the patients are using the social networking support the state anger increases and environment increase.

Table 84

Moderating Effect of Active Focused Coping Strategies on Relationship of Anger Control-In with Self-Acceptance, Positive Relations with others and Autonomy (n = 500)

Variables	Self-acceptance		Positive relations with others		Autonomy	
	ΔR^2	β	ΔR^2	β	ΔR^2	β
Step 1						
Anger control-In		.081		-.07		-.12*
Active focused coping		.19**		-.14*		.07
Step 2	.01*		.06***		.012*	
Anger control-In * Active focused coping		-.13*		-.28***		.12*
R^2	.04**		.08***		.02*	

*** $p < .001$, ** $p < .01$, * $p < .05$.

Table 84 illustrates moderation analysis for active focused coping strategies in the relationship between anger control-In and psychological well-being (Self-Acceptance, positive relations with others and autonomy). Active focused coping strategies are acting as a moderator for the relationship of anger control-In with Self-Acceptance, positive relations with others and autonomy. These added additional 1% variance is explained by the relationship (self-acceptance and Anger control-In) which is moderated by active focused coping strategies. It also added additional 6% variance is explained by the relationship (positive relations with others and anger control-in) which is moderated by active focused coping strategies. It also added additional 12% variance is explained by the autonomy and anger control-in which is moderated by active focused coping strategies. The moderating effect is further explained through mod graphs.

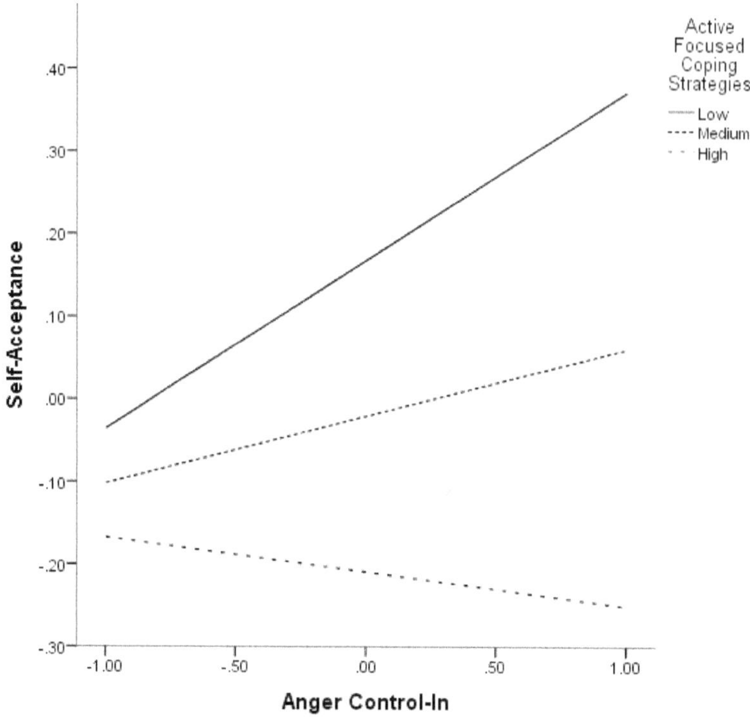

Figure 69. Active focused coping strategies as a moderator between self-acceptance and anger control - in

The correlation of anger control-in with personal physical functioning is moderated by the active focused coping strategies. When the active focused coping strategies are increasingly used by the patients, the relationship between anger control-in and self-acceptance is positive, which means that in case if the patients are using the active focused coping strategies the anger control-in increases and self-acceptance also increases.

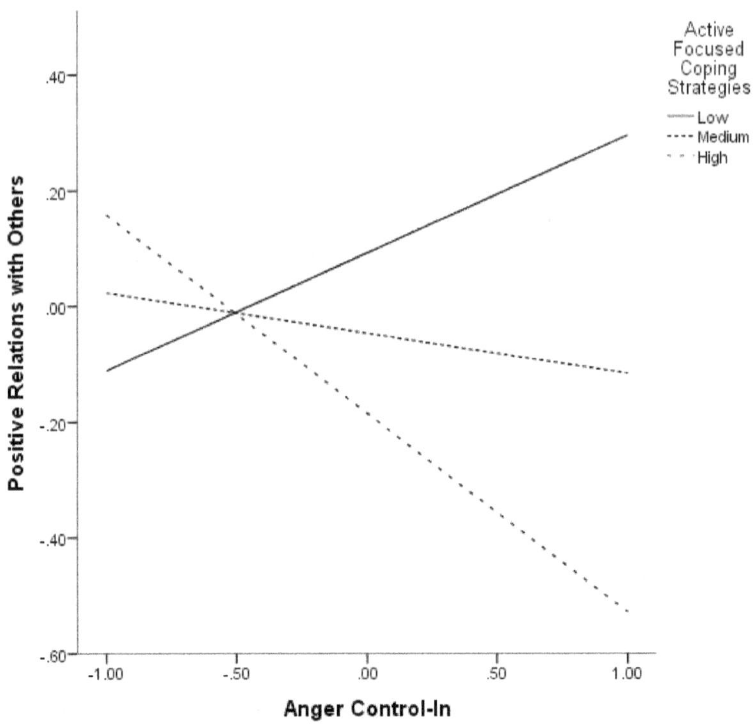

Figure 70. Active focused coping strategies as a moderator between positive relations with others and anger control - in

The correlation of anger control-in with positive relations with others is moderated by the active focused coping strategies. When the active focused coping strategies are increasingly used by the patients, the relationship between anger control-in and positive relations with others is negative, which means that in case if the patients are using the active focused coping strategies the anger control-in increases and positive relations with others decreases.

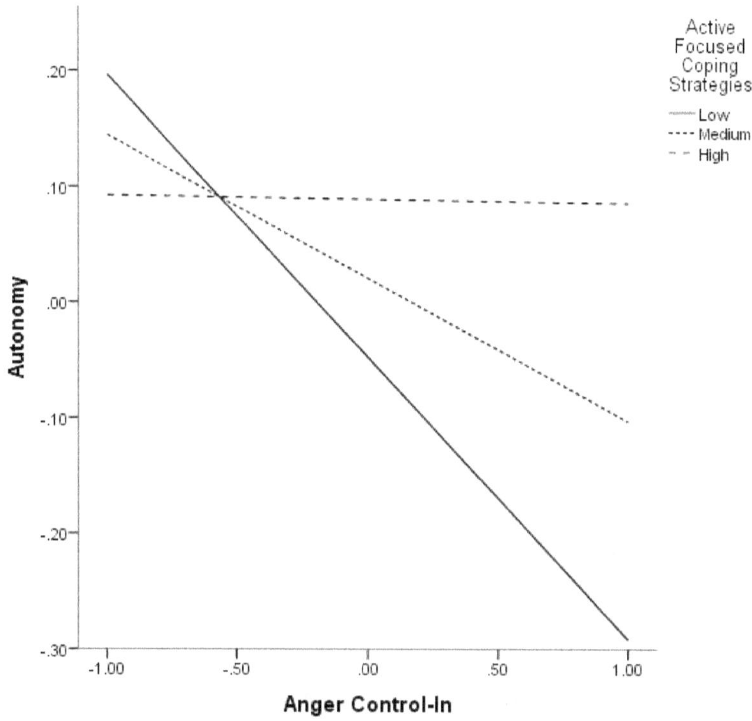

Figure 71. Active focused coping strategies as a moderator between autonomy and anger control - in

The correlation of anger control-in with autonomy is moderated by the active focused coping strategies. When the active focused coping strategies are increasingly used by the patients, the relationship between anger control-in and autonomy, which means that in case if the patients are using the active focused coping strategies the anger control-in increases and autonomy also increases.

Table 85

Moderating Effect of active distracting coping strategies on Relationship of Anger control-In with self-acceptance, positive relations with others and autonomy (n = 500)

Variables	Self-acceptance		Positive relations with others		Autonomy	
	ΔR^2	β	ΔR^2	β	ΔR^2	β
Step 1						
Anger control-In		.08		-.14*		-.10*
Active distracting coping		-.04		.06		.07
Step 2	.00		.00		.00	
Anger control-In * Active distracting coping		.05		.06		-.00
R^2	.01		.03**		.02*	

***p < .001, ** p < .01, * p < .05.

Table 85 illustrates moderation analysis for active distracting coping strategies in the relationship between anger control-In and psychological well-being (Self-Acceptance, positive relations with others and autonomy). Active distracting coping strategies are not acting as a moderator for the relationship of anger control-In with Self-Acceptance, positive relations with others and autonomy.

Table 86

Moderating Effect of Avoidance Focused Coping Strategies on Relationship of Anger Control-In with Self-Acceptance, Positive Relations with Others and Autonomy (n = 500)

Variables	Self-acceptance		Positive relations with others		Autonomy	
	ΔR^2	β	ΔR^2	β	ΔR^2	β
Step 1						
Anger control-In		.03		-.11*		-.06
Avoidance focused coping strategies		-.16		-.10		.22*
Step 2	.00		.07***		.02*	
Anger control-In * Avoidance focused coping strategies		-.69		-.38***		.19*
R^2	.01		.11***		.03*	

***$p < .001$, ** $p < .01$, * $p < .05$.

Table 86 illustrates moderation analysis for Avoidance focused coping strategies in the relationship between anger control-In and psychological well-being (Self-Acceptance, positive relations with others and autonomy). Avoidance focused coping strategies are acting as a moderator for the relationship of anger control-In with positive relations with others and autonomy. These added additional 7% variance is explained by the relationship (positive relations with others and anger control-in) which is moderated by Avoidance focused coping strategies. It also added additional 2% variance is explained by the autonomy and anger control-in which is moderated by Avoidance focused coping strategies. The moderating effect is further explained through mod graphs.

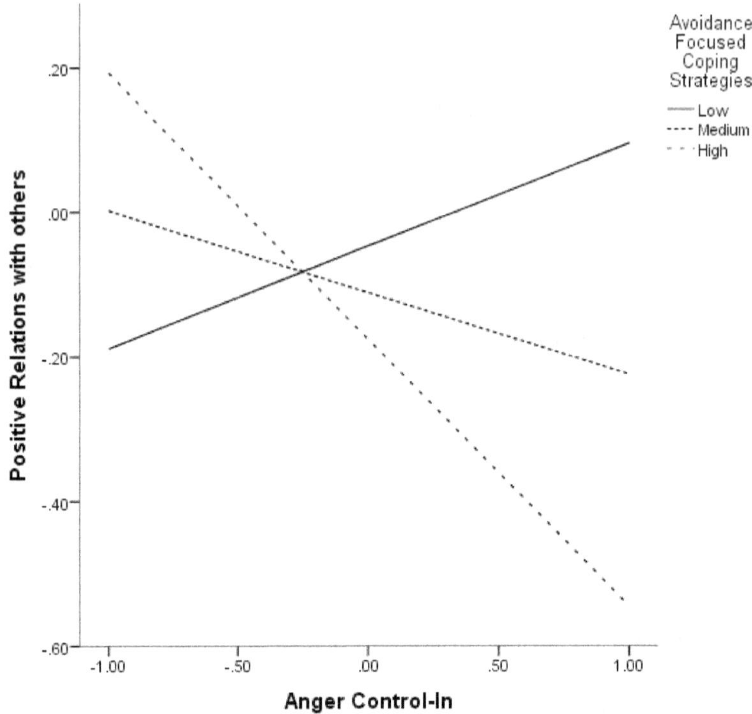

Figure 72. Avoidance focused coping strategies as a moderator between positive relations with others and anger control - in

The correlation of anger control-in with positive relations with others is moderated by the avoidance focused coping strategies. When the avoidance focused coping strategies are increasingly used by the patients, the relationship between anger control-in and positive relations with others is negative, which means that in case if the patients are using the avoidance focused coping strategies the anger control-in increases and positive relations with others decreases.

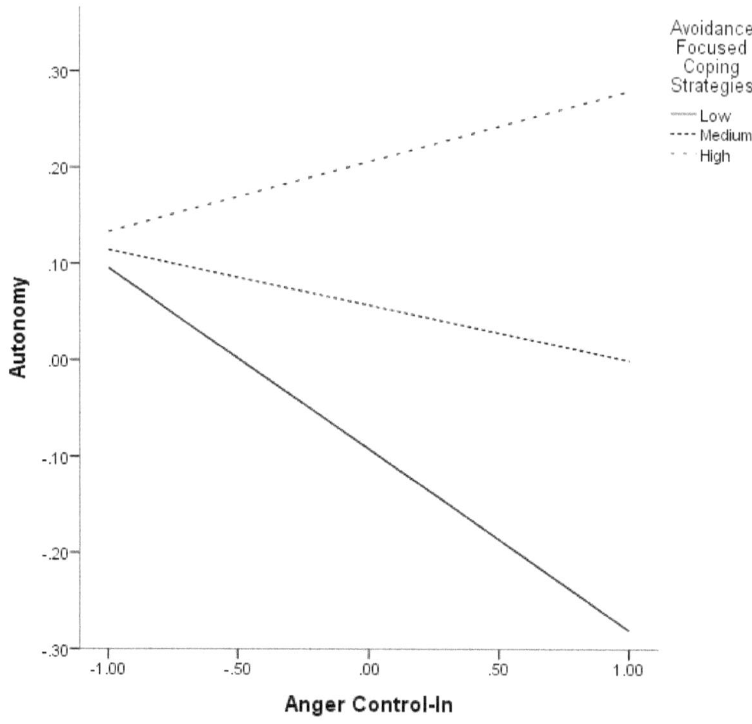

Figure 73. Avoidance focused coping strategies as a moderator between autonomy and anger control - in

The correlation of anger control-in with autonomy is moderated by the avoidance focused coping strategies. When the avoidance focused coping strategies are increasingly used by the patients, the relationship between anger control-in and autonomy is negative, which means that in case if the patients are using the avoidance focused coping strategies the anger control-in increases and autonomy decreases.

Table 87

Moderating Effect of Religious Focused Coping Strategies on Relationship of Anger Control-In with Self-Acceptance, Positive Relations with Others and Autonomy (n = 500)

Variables	Self-acceptance		Positive relations with others		Autonomy	
	$\triangle R^2$	β	$\triangle R^2$	β	$\triangle R^2$	β
Step 1						
Anger control-In		.10*		-.12*		-.17**
Religious focused coping strategies		-.03		-.07		-.08*
Step 2	.04***		.08***		.03**	
Anger control-In * Religious focused coping strategies		-.17***		-.25***		.15**
R^2	.05***		.12***		.04**	

***$p < .001$, ** $p < .01$, * $p < .05$.

Table 87 illustrates moderation analysis for Religious focused coping strategies in the relationship between anger control-In and psychological well-being (Self-Acceptance, positive relations with others and autonomy). Religious focused coping strategies are acting as a moderator for the relationship of anger control-In with positive relations with others and autonomy. These added additional 4% variance is explained by the relationship (self-acceptance and anger control-in) which is moderated by religious focused coping strategies. These added additional 8% variance is explained by the relationship (positive relations with others and anger control-in) which is moderated by religious focused coping strategies. It also added additional 3% variance is explained by the autonomy and anger control-in which is moderated by religious focused coping strategies. The moderating effect is further explained through mod graphs.

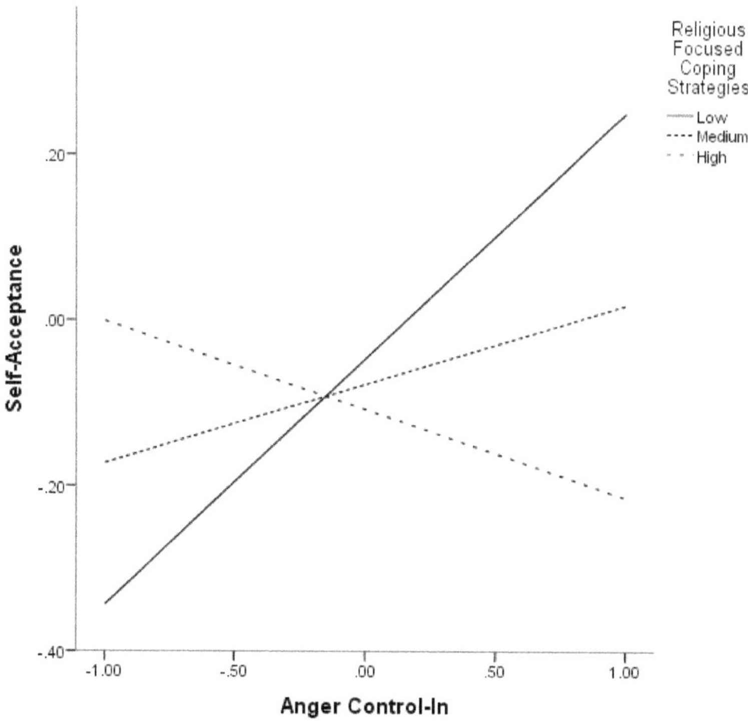

Figure 74. Religious focused coping strategies as a moderator between self-acceptance and anger control - in

The correlation of anger control-in with self-acceptance by the religious focused coping strategies. When the religious focused coping strategies are increasingly used by the patients, the relationship between anger control-in and self-acceptance is negative, which means that in case if the patients are using the religious focused coping strategies the anger control-in increases and self-acceptance decreases.

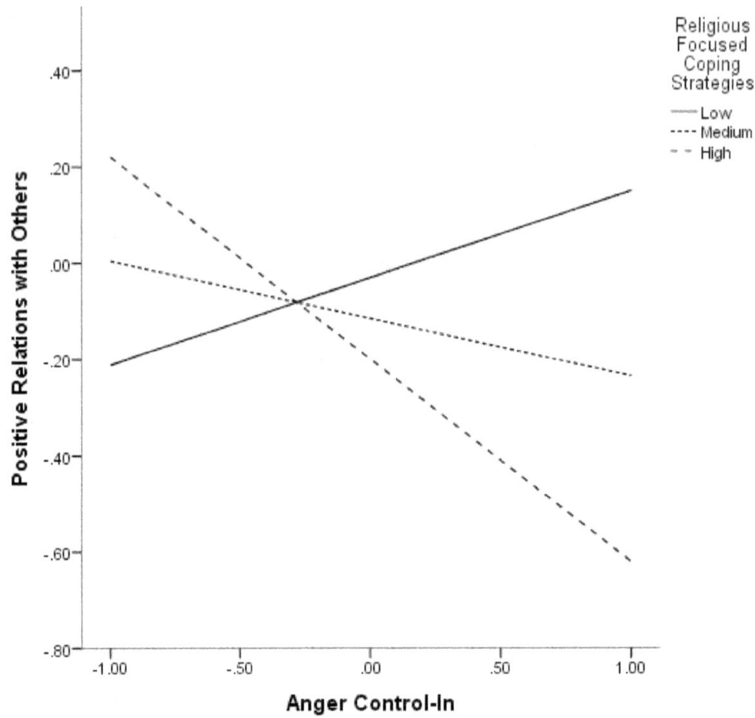

Figure 75. Religious focused coping strategies as a moderator between Positive relations with others and anger control - in

The correlation of anger control-in with positive relations with others is moderated by the religious focused coping strategies. When the religious focused coping strategies are increasingly used by the patients, the relationship between anger control-in and positive relations with others is negative, which means that in case if the patients are using the religious focused coping strategies the anger control-in increases and positive relations with others decreases.

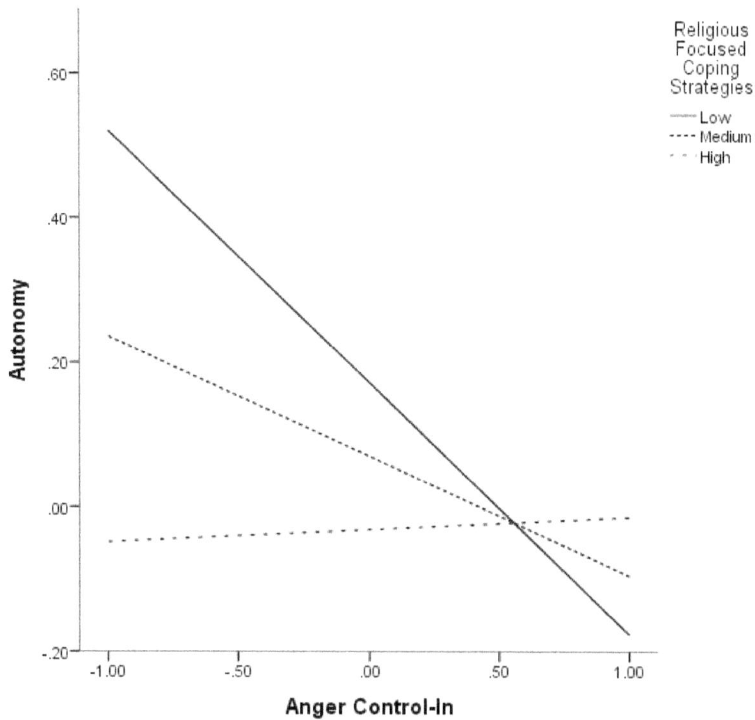

Figure 76. Religious focused coping strategies as a moderator between autonomy and anger control - in

The correlation of anger control-in with autonomy is moderated by the religious focused coping strategies. When the religious focused coping strategies are increasingly used by the patients, the relationship between anger control-in and autonomy is negative, which means that in case if the patients are using the religious focused coping strategies the anger control-in increases and autonomy decreases.

Table 88

Moderating Effect of Informational Support on Relationship of Anger control-In with Self-Acceptance, Positive Relations with Others and Autonomy (n = 500)

Variables	Self-acceptance		Positive relations with others		Autonomy	
	$\triangle R^2$	β	$\triangle R^2$	β	$\triangle R^2$	β
Step 1						
Anger control-In		.09*		-.11*		-.12*
Informational Support		-.18**		-.22***		.22***
Step 2	.00		.01*		.01	
Anger control-In * Informational Support		.07		.12*		-.09
R^2	.04**		.08***		.06***	

$***p < .001, ** p < .01, * p < .05.$

Table 88 illustrates moderation analysis for Informational support in the relationship between anger control-In and psychological well-being (Self-Acceptance, positive relations with others and autonomy). Informational support is acting as a moderator for the relationship of anger control-In with positive relations with others. These added additional 1% variance is explained by the relationship (self-acceptance and anger control-in) which is moderated by informational support. The moderating effect is further explained through mod graphs.

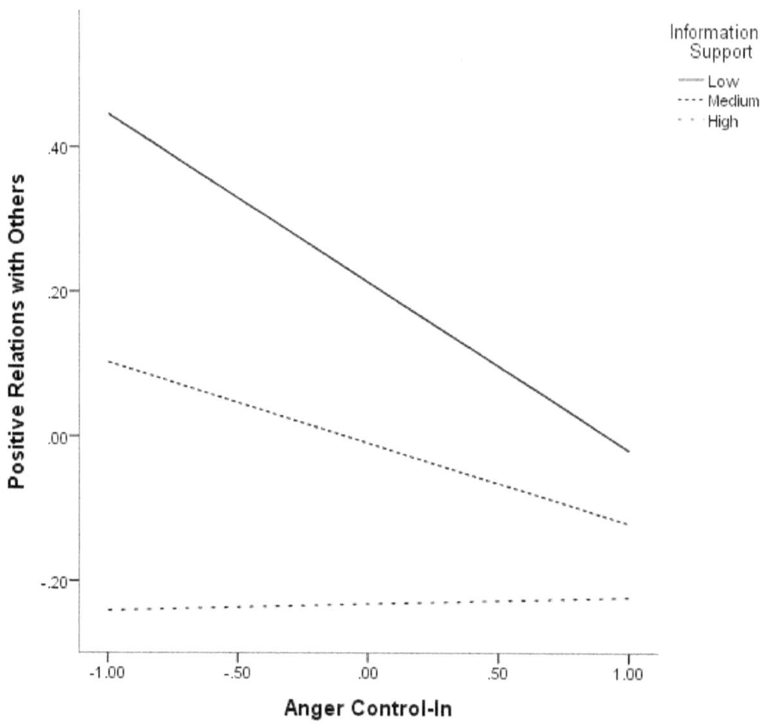

Figure 77. Informational Support as a moderator between positive relations with others and anger control - in

The correlation of anger control-in and positive relations with others is moderated by the informational support. When the informational support is increasingly used by the patients, the relationship between anger control-in and positive relations with others is negative, which means that in case if the patients are using the informational support the anger control-in increases and positive relations with others decreases.

Table 89

Moderating Effect of Tangible Support on Relationship of Anger Control-In with Self-Acceptance, Positive Relations with Others and Autonomy (n = 500)

Variables	Self-acceptance		Positive relations with others		Autonomy	
	$\triangle R^2$	β	$\triangle R^2$	β	$\triangle R^2$	β
Step 1						
Anger control-In		.08		-.14**		-.10*
Tangible Support		-.19***		-.26***		.14**
Step 2	.01		.00		.00	
Anger control-In * Tangible Support		-.07		-.04		.06
R^2	.04**		.09***		.03**	

***$p < .001$, ** $p < .01$, * $p < .05$.

Table 89 illustrates moderation analysis for Tangible support in the relationship between anger control-In and psychological well-being (Self-Acceptance, positive relations with others and autonomy). Tangible support is not acting as a moderator for the relationship of anger control-In with positive relations with others.

Table 90

Moderating Effect of Emotional Support on Relationship of Anger Control-In with Self-Acceptance, Positive Relations with Others and Autonomy (n = 500)

Variables	Self-acceptance		Positive relations with others		Autonomy	
	$\triangle R^2$	β	$\triangle R^2$	β	$\triangle R^2$	β
Step 1						
Anger control-In		.10*		-.12**		-.13*
Emotional Support		-.06		.05		.13*
Step 2	.02**		.03**		.00	
Anger control-In * Emotional Support		.18**		.25**		-.09
R^2	.03**		.05***		.04**	

***$p < .001$, ** $p < .01$, * $p < .05$.

Table 90 illustrates moderation analysis for Emotional support in the relationship between anger control-In and psychological well-being (Self-Acceptance, positive relations with others and autonomy). Emotional support is acting as a moderator for the relationship of anger control-In with self-acceptance and positive relations with others. These added additional 2% variance is explained by the relationship (self-acceptance and anger control-in) which is moderated by emotional support. It also added additional 3% variance is explained by the relationship (positive relations with others and anger control-in) which is moderated by emotional support. The moderating effect is further explained through mod graphs.

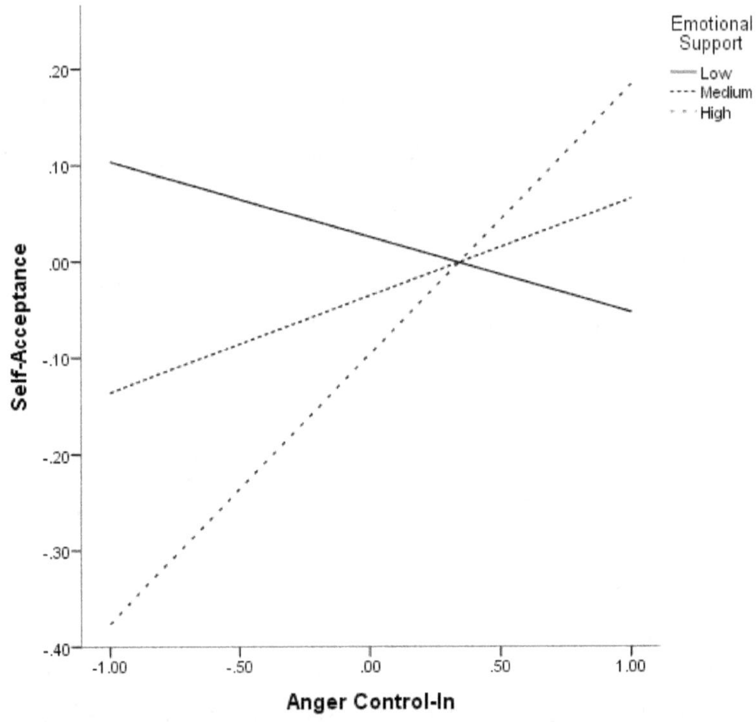

Figure 78. Emotional Support as a moderator between self-acceptance and anger control - in

The correlation of anger control-in with self-acceptance is moderated by the emotional support. When the emotional support is increasingly used by the patients, the relationship between anger control-in and self-acceptance is positive, which means that in case if the patients are using the emotional support the anger control-in increases and self-acceptance also increases.

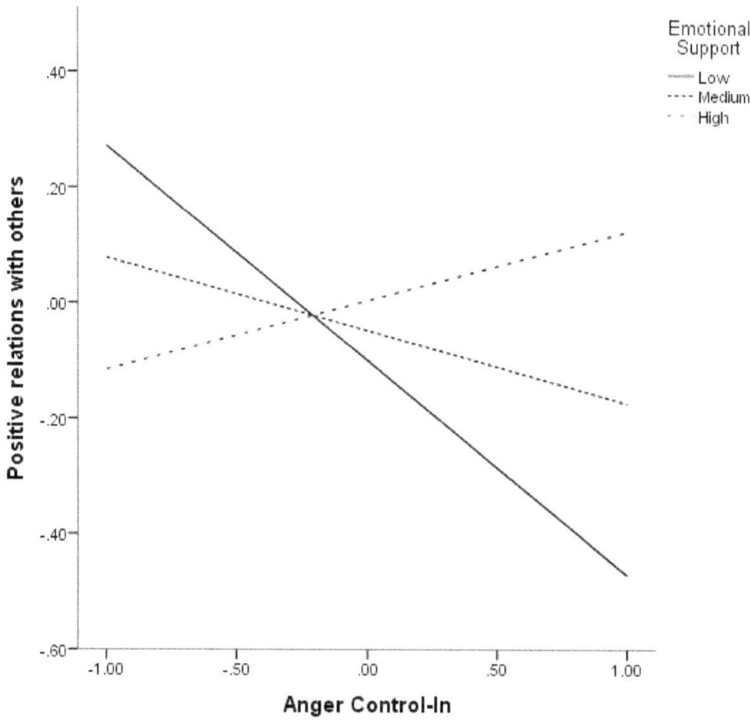

Figure 79. Emotional Support as a moderator between positive relations with others and anger control - in

The correlation of anger control-in with positive relations with others is moderated by the emotional support. When the emotional support is increasingly used by the patients, the relationship between anger control-in and positive relations with others is positive, which means that in case if the patients are using the emotional support the anger control-in increases and positive relations with others also increases.

Table 91

Moderating Effect of Esteem Support on Relationship of Anger Control-In with Self-Acceptance, Positive Relations with Others and Autonomy (n = 500)

Variables	Self-acceptance		Positive relations with others		Autonomy	
	$\triangle R^2$	β	$\triangle R^2$	β	$\triangle R^2$	β
Step 1						
Anger control-In		.08		-.14*		-.12*
Esteem Support		-.08		-.03		.15*
Step 2	.01*		.01		.00	
Anger control-In * Esteem Support		.14*		.10		-.06
R^2	.03**		.03*		.04**	

***p < .001, ** p < .01, * p < .05.

Table 91 illustrates moderation analysis for Esteem support in the relationship between anger control-In and psychological well-being (Self-Acceptance, positive relations with others and autonomy). Esteem support is acting as a moderator for the relationship of anger control-In with self-acceptance. These added additional 1% variance is explained by the relationship (self-acceptance and anger control-in) which is moderated by esteem support. The moderating effect is further explained through mod graph.

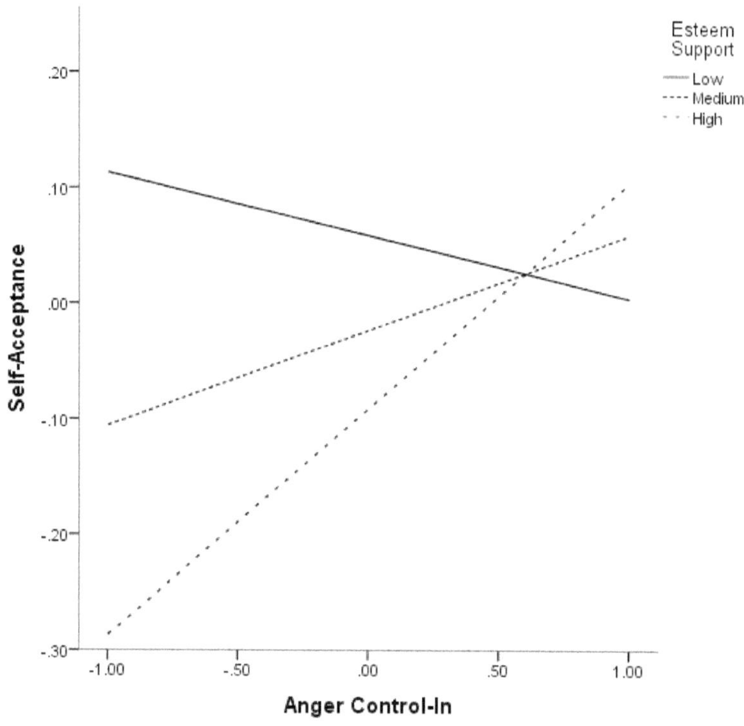

Figure 80. Esteem Support as a moderator between self-acceptance and anger control - in

The correlation of anger control-in with self-acceptance is moderated by the esteem support. When the esteem support is increasingly used by the patients, the relationship between anger control-in and self-acceptance is positive, which means that in case if the patients are using the esteem support the anger control-in increases and self-acceptance also increases.

Table 92

Moderating Effect of Social Network Support on Relationship of Anger Control-In with Self-Acceptance, Positive Relations with Others and Autonomy (n = 500)

Variables	Self-acceptance		Positive relations with others		Autonomy	
	$\triangle R^2$	β	$\triangle R^2$	β	$\triangle R^2$	β
Step 1						
Anger control-In		.08		-.14*		-.10
Social Network Support		-.14**		-.04		.21
Step 2	.01		.00		.00	
Anger control-In * Social Network Support		.09		-.02		-.01
R^2	.03*		.02		.05***	

***p < .001, ** p < .01, * p < .05.

Table 92 illustrates moderation analysis for social networking support in the relationship between anger control-In and psychological well-being (Self-Acceptance, positive relations with others and autonomy). Social networking support is not acting as a moderator for the relationship of anger control-In with self-acceptance, positive relations with others and autonomy.

Table 93

Moderating Effect of active focused coping strategies on Relationship of Anger Control-In with Psychological Health, Social Relationships and Environment (n = 500)

Variables	Psychological health		Social relationships		Environment	
	$\triangle R^2$	β	$\triangle R^2$	β	$\triangle R^2$	β
Step 1						
Anger control-In		-2.20**		-2.07*		-4.73**
Active focused coping		.42		4.08**		7.28*
Step 2	.15***		.012**		.02**	
Anger control-In * Active focused coping		.28**		.27**		.61**
R^2	.01**		.35***		.42***	

***p < .001, ** p < .01, * p < .05.

Table 93 illustrates moderation analysis for active coping strategies in the relationship between anger control-In and quality of life (Psychological functioning, Social relationships and Environment). Active focused coping strategies are acting as a moderator for the relationship of anger control-In with Physical functioning, Psychological functioning, Social relationships and Environment. These added additional 15% variance is explained by the relationship (Psychological functioning and anger control-in) which is moderated by active focused coping strategies. It also added additional 12% variance is explained by the social relationships and anger control-in which is moderated by active focused coping strategies. It also added additional 2% variance is explained by the relationship (environment and Anger control-in) which is moderated by active focused coping strategies. The moderating effect is further explained through mod graphs.

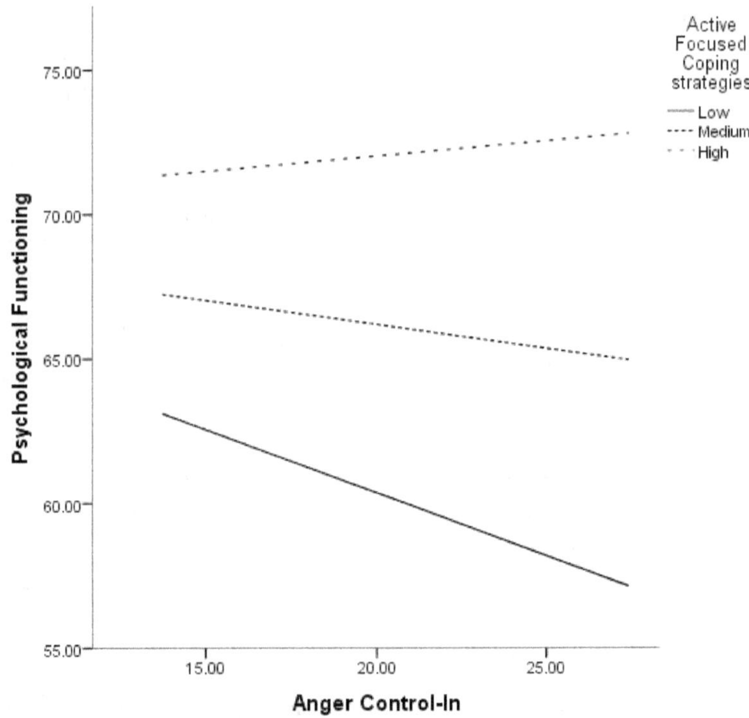

Figure 81. Active focused coping strategies as a moderator between psychological functioning and anger control - in

The correlation of anger control-in with personal psychological functioning is moderated by the active focused coping strategies. When the active focused coping strategies are increasingly used by the patients, the relationship between anger control-in and physical functioning is negative, which means that in case if the patients are using the active focused coping strategies the anger control-in increases and psychological functioning also decreases.

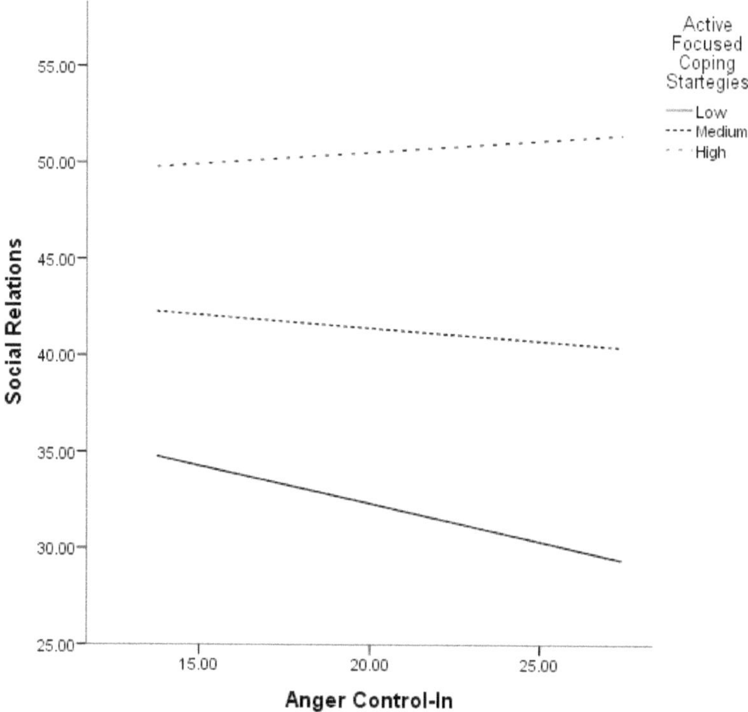

Figure 82. Active focused coping strategies as a moderator between social relations and anger control - in

The correlation of anger control-in with social relationship is moderated by the active focused coping strategies. When the active focused coping strategies are increasingly used by the patients, the relationship between anger control-in and social relationship is positive, which means that in case if the patients are using the active focused coping strategies the anger control-in increases and social relationship also increases.

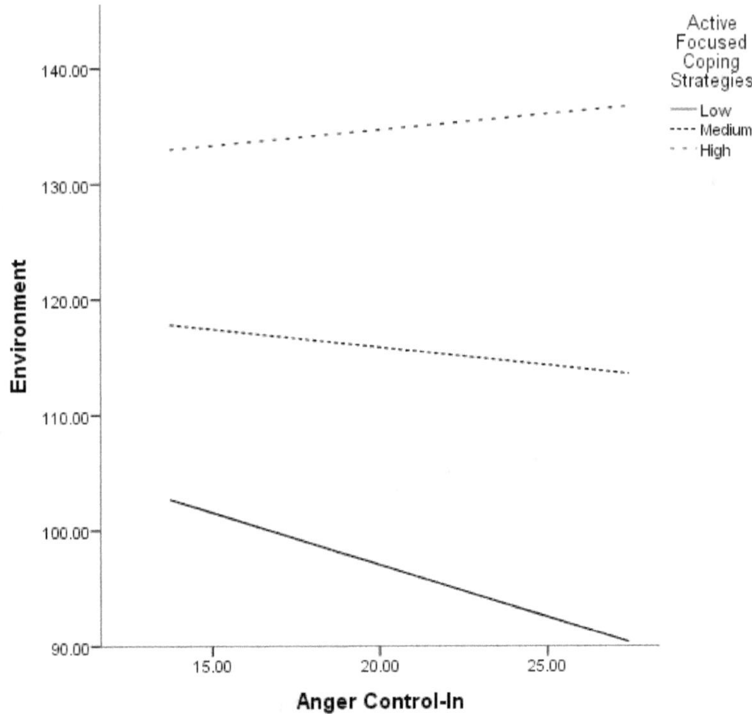

Figure 83. Active focused coping strategies as a moderator between environment and anger control - in

The correlation of anger control-in with environment is moderated by the active focused coping strategies. When the active focused coping strategies are increasingly used by the patients, the relationship between anger control-in and environment is positive, which means that in case if the patients are using the active focused coping strategies the anger control-in increases and environment also increases.

Table 94

Moderating Effect of active distracting coping strategies on Relationship of Anger Control-In with Psychological Health, Social Relationships and Environment (n = 500)

Variables	Psychological health		Social relationships		Environment	
	ΔR^2	β	ΔR^2	β	ΔR^2	β
Step 1						
Anger control-In		-1.55*		-2.00*		-4.54***
Active distracting coping		2.15***		2.61***		12.95***
Step 2	.00		.00		.00	
Anger control-In * Active distracting coping		.38		-.05		.08
R^2	.05***		.07***		.37***	

***$p < .001$, ** $p < .01$, * $p < .05$.

Table 94 illustrates moderation analysis for active distracting coping strategies in the relationship between anger control-In and quality of life (Psychological functioning, Social relationships and Environment). Active distracting coping strategies are not acting as a moderator for the relationship of anger control-In with Physical functioning, Psychological functioning, Social relationships and Environment.

Table 95

Moderating Effect of avoidance focused coping strategies on Relationship of Anger Control-In with Psychological Health, Social Relationships and Environment (n = 500)

Variables	Psychological health		Social relationships		Environment	
	$\triangle R^2$	β	$\triangle R^2$	β	$\triangle R^2$	β
Step 1						
Anger control-In		1.43*		.511		4.80***
Avoidance focused coping		12.86***		10.57***		37.78***
Step 2	.06***		.04***		.13***	
Anger control-In * Avoidance focused coping		5.46***		4.55***		14.87***
R^2	.18***		.13***		.42***	

*** $p < .001$, ** $p < .01$, * $p < .05$.

Table 95 illustrates moderation analysis for avoidance focused coping strategies in the relationship between anger control-In and quality of life (Psychological functioning, Social relationships and Environment). Avoidance focused coping strategies are acting as a moderator for the relationship of anger control-In with Physical functioning, Psychological functioning, Social relationships and Environment. These added additional 6% variance is explained by the relationship (Psychological functioning and anger control-in) which is moderated by avoidance focused coping strategies. It also added additional 4% variance is explained by the social relationships and anger control-in which is moderated by avoidance focused coping strategies. It also added additional 13% variance is explained by the relationship (environment and Anger control-in) which is moderated by avoidance focused coping strategies. The moderating effect is further explained through mod graphs.

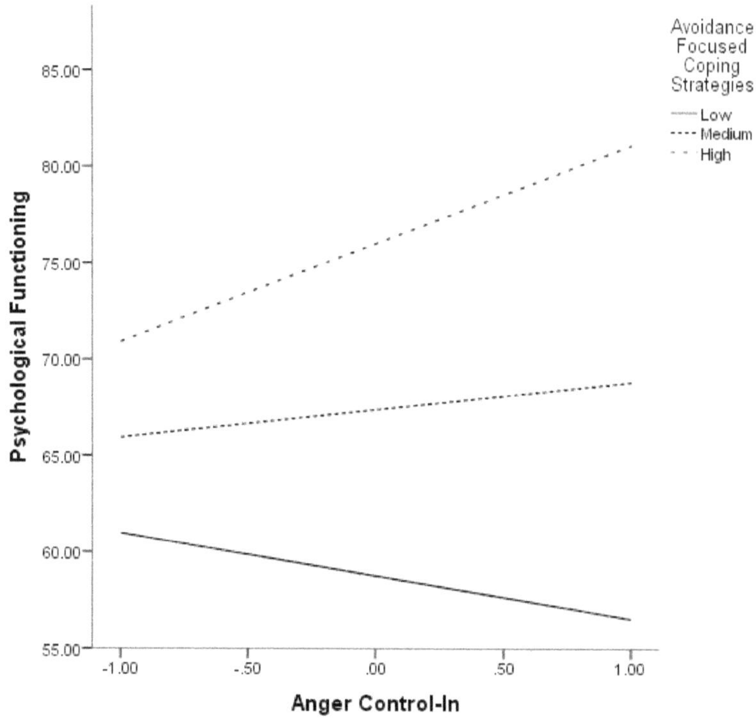

Figure 84. Avoidance focused coping strategies as a moderator between psychological functioning and anger control - in

The correlation of anger control-in with psychological functioning is moderated by the avoidance focused coping strategies. When the avoidance focused coping strategies are increasingly used by the patients, the relationship between anger control-in and psychological functioning is positive, which means that in case if the patients are using the avoidance focused coping strategies the anger control-in increases and psychological functioning also increases.

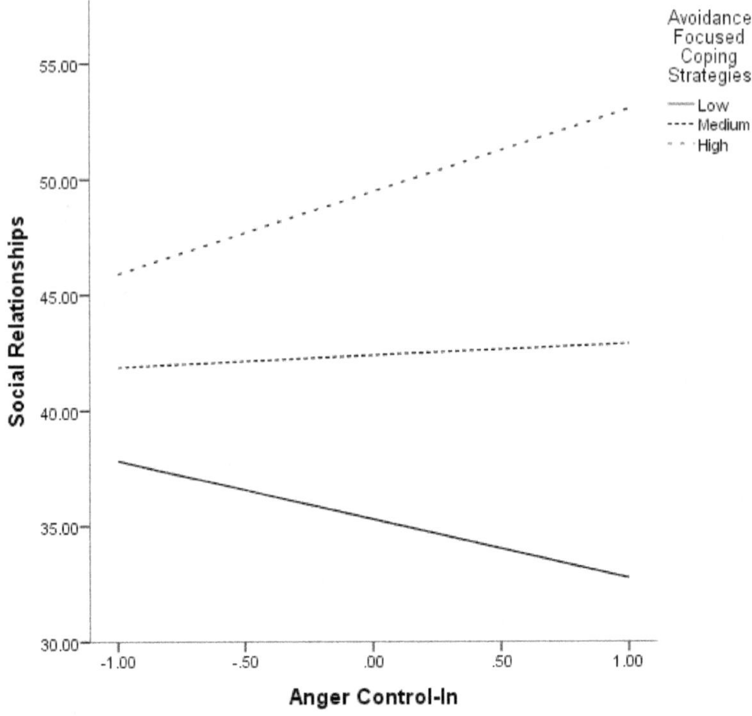

Figure 85. Avoidance focused coping strategies as a moderator between social relationships and anger control – in

The correlation of anger control-in with social relationships is moderated by the avoidance focused coping strategies. When the avoidance focused coping strategies are increasingly used by the patients, the relationship between anger control-in and social relationships is positive, which means that in case if the patients are using the avoidance focused coping strategies the anger control-in increases and social relationships also increases.

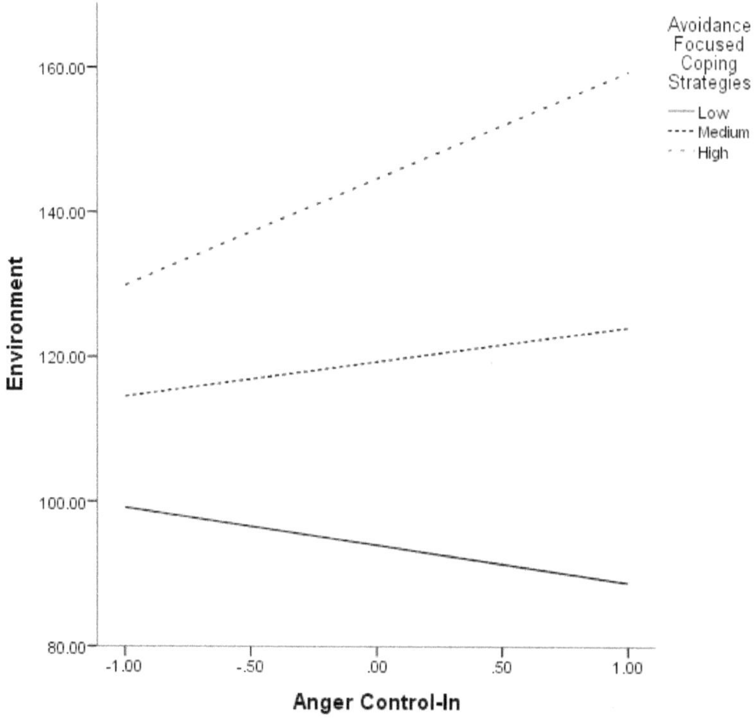

Figure 86: Avoidance focused coping strategies as a moderator between environment and anger control - in

The correlation of anger control-in with environment is moderated by the avoidance focused coping strategies. When the avoidance focused coping strategies are increasingly used by the patients, the relationship between anger control-in and environment is positive, which means that in case if the patients are using the avoidance focused coping strategies the anger control-in increases and environment also increases.

Table 96

Moderating Effect of Religious focused coping strategies on Relationship of Anger Control-In with Psychological Health, Social Relationships and Environment (n = 500)

Variables	Psychological health		Social relationships		Environment	
	ΔR^2	β	ΔR^2	β	ΔR^2	β
Step 1						
Anger control-In		-.73		.87		3.14*
Religious focused coping		1.47*		5.34***		14.33***
Step 2	.00		.01*		.01*	
Anger control-In * Religious focused coping		-.41		-1.29*		-2.31*
R^2	.02*		.17***		.33***	

***$p < .001$, ** $p < .01$, * $p < .05$.

Table 96 illustrates moderation analysis for religious focused coping strategies in the relationship between anger control-In and quality of life (Psychological functioning, Social relationships and Environment). Religious focused coping strategies are acting as a moderator for the relationship of anger control-In with Social relationships and Environment. These added additional 1% variance is explained by the social relationships and anger control-in which is moderated by religious focused coping strategies. It also added additional 1% variance is explained by the relationship (environment and Anger control-in) which is moderated by religious focused coping strategies. The moderating effect is further explained through mod graphs.

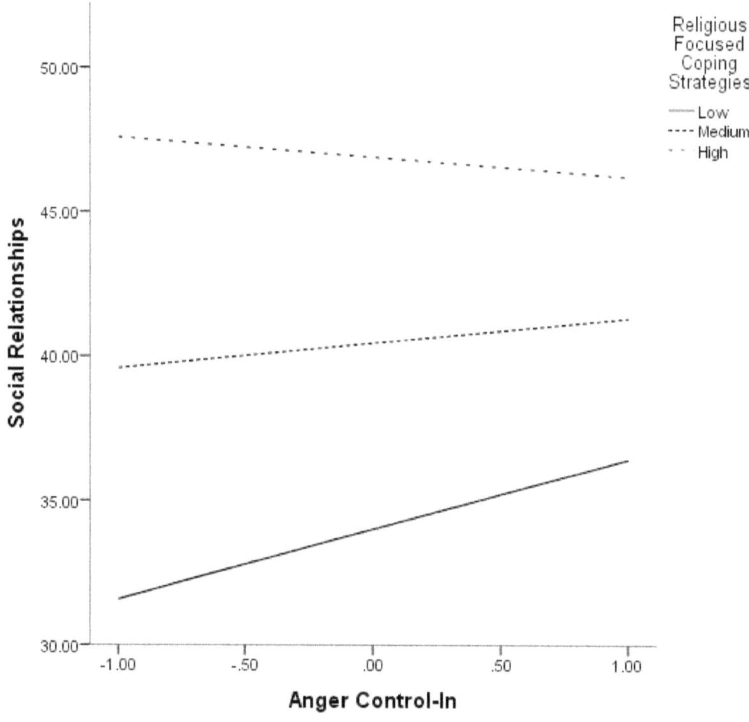

Figure 87: Religious focused coping strategies as a moderator between social relationships and anger control - in

The correlation of anger control-in with social relationships is moderated by the religious focused coping strategies. When the religious focused coping strategies are increasingly used by the patients, the relationship between anger control-in and social relationships is positive, which means that in case if the patients are using the religious focused coping strategies the anger control-in increases and social relationships also increases.

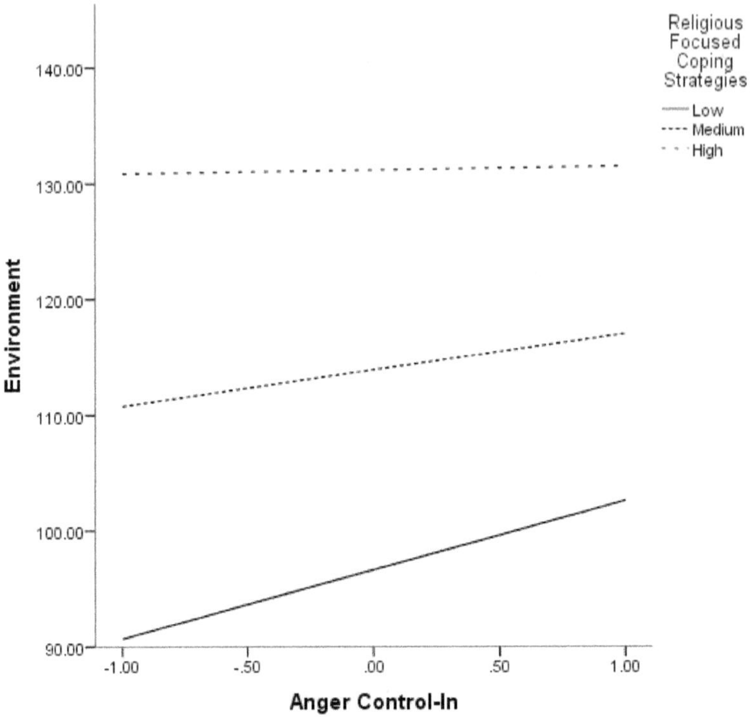

Figure 88. Religious focused coping strategies as a moderator between environment and anger control - in

The correlation of anger control-in with environment is moderated by the religious focused coping strategies. When the religious focused coping strategies are increasingly used by the patients, the relationship between anger control-in and environment is positive, which means that in case if the patients are using the religious focused coping strategies the anger control-in increases and environment also increases.

Table 97

Moderating Effect of Informational Support on Relationship of Anger Control-In with Psychological Health, Social Relationships and Environment (n = 500)

Variables	Psychological health		Social relationships		Environment	
	$\triangle R^2$	β	$\triangle R^2$	β	$\triangle R^2$	β
Step 1						
Anger control-In		-1.81*		-2.31**		-5.17***
Informational Support		2.09*		4.91***		12.31***
Step 2	.01		.00		.00	
Anger control-In * Informational Support		-1.34		-.31		-1.76
R^2	.03**		.12***		.21***	

***$p < .001$, ** $p < .01$, * $p < .05$.

Table 97 illustrates moderation analysis for informational support in the relationship between anger control-In and quality of life (Psychological functioning, Social relationships and Environment). Informational support is not acting as a moderator for the relationship of anger control-In with psychological functioning, Social relationships and Environment.

Table 98

Moderating Effect of Tangible Support on Relationship of Anger Control-In with Psychological Health, Social Relationships and Environment (n = 500)

Variables	Psychological health $\triangle R^2$	β	Social relationships $\triangle R^2$	β	Environment $\triangle R^2$	β
Step 1						
Anger control-In		-1.54*		-1.96*		-4.20**
Tangible Support		4.82***		5.82***		14.28***
Step 2	.00		.00		.00	
Anger control-In * Tangible Support		-.45		.08		.59
R^2	.12***		.17***		.27***	

***p < .001, ** p < .01, * p < .05.

Table 98 illustrates moderation analysis for tangible support in the relationship between anger control-In and quality of life (Psychological functioning, Social relationships and Environment). Tangible support is not acting as a moderator for the relationship of anger control-In with psychological functioning, Social relationships and Environment.

Table 99

Moderating Effect of Emotional Support on Relationship of Anger Control-In with Psychological Health, Social Relationships and Environment (n = 500)

Variables	Psychological health		Social relationships		Environment	
	$\triangle R^2$	β	$\triangle R^2$	β	$\triangle R^2$	β
Step 1						
Anger control-In		-2.76***		-3.30***		-8.03***
Emotional Support		.63***		7.32***		21.88***
Step 2	.00		.00		.01*	
Anger control-In * Emotional Support		.44		.34		2.74*
R^2	.20***		.24***		.57***	

***$p < .001$, ** $p < .01$, * $p < .05$.

Table 99 illustrates moderation analysis for emotional support in the relationship between anger control-In and quality of life (Psychological functioning, Social relationships and Environment). Emotional support is acting as a moderator for the relationship of anger control-In with environment. These added additional 1% variance is explained by the relationship (environment and Anger control-in) which is moderated by emotional support. The moderating effect is further explained through mod graph.

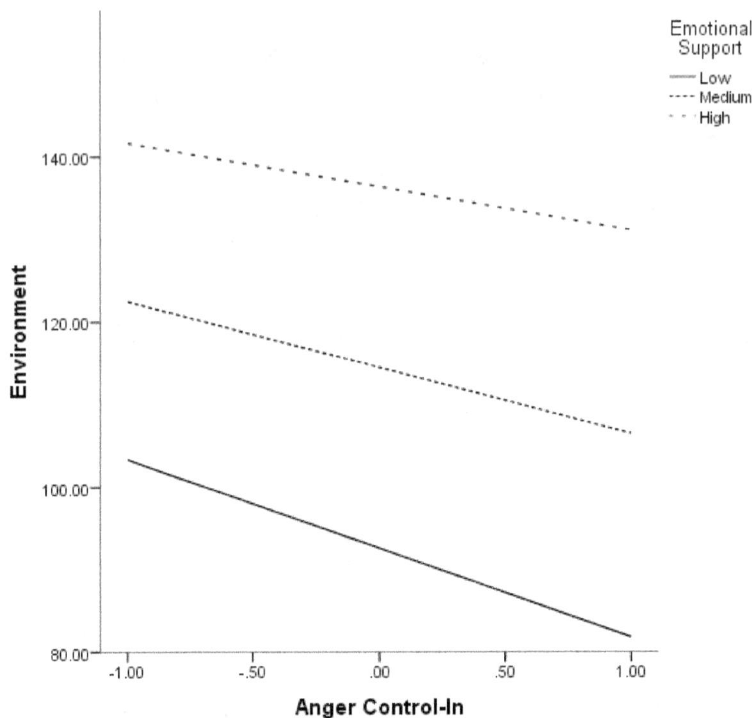

Figure 89. Emotional Support as a moderator between environment and anger control - in

The correlation of anger control-in with environment is moderated by the emotional support. When the emotional support is increasingly used by the patients, the relationship between anger control-in and environment is negative, which means that in case if the patients are using the emotional support the anger control-in increases and environment decreases.

Table 100

Moderating Effect of Esteem Support on Relationship of Anger Control-In with Psychological Health, Social Relationships and Environment (n = 500)

	Psychological health		Social relationships		Environment	
Variables	$\triangle R^2$	β	$\triangle R^2$	β	$\triangle R^2$	β
Step 1						
Anger control-In		-2.56***		-3.34***		-7.47***
Esteem Support		6.03***		8.25***		20.05***
Step 2	.00		.00		.00	
Anger control-In * Esteem Support		.66		-.27		-.44
R^2	.17***		.31***		.51***	

***$p < .001$, ** $p < .01$, * $p < .05$.

Table 100 illustrates moderation analysis for esteem support in the relationship between anger control-In and quality of life (Psychological functioning, Social relationships and Environment). Esteem support is not acting as a moderator for the relationship of anger control-In with psychological functioning, social relationships and environment.

Table 101

Moderating effect of social network support on relationship of anger control-in with psychological health, social Relationships and Environment (n = 500)

Variables	Psychological health		Social relationships		Environment	
	ΔR^2	β	ΔR^2	β	ΔR^2	β
Step 1						
Anger control-In		-1.10**		-2.46***		-5.51***
Social Network Support		9.19***		9.31***		24.78***
Step 2	.00		.01**		.02***	
Anger control-In * Social Network Support		-1.10		-1.99**		-5.12***
R^2	.38***		.38***		.75***	

***p < .001, ** p < .01, * p < .05.

Table 101 illustrates moderation analysis for esteem support in the relationship between anger control-In and quality of life (Psychological functioning, Social relationships and Environment). Esteem support is not acting as a moderator for the relationship of anger control-In with psychological functioning, social relationships and environment.

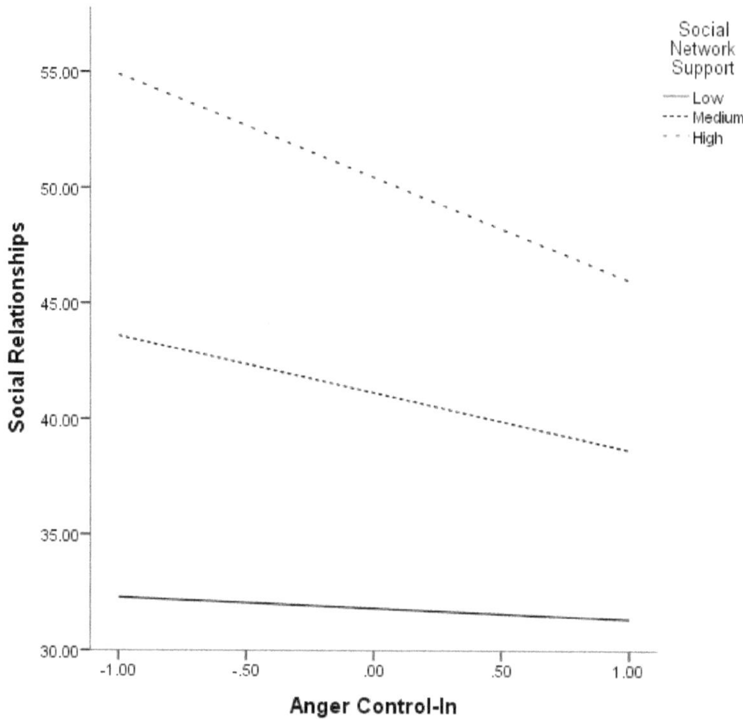

Figure 90. Social Network Support as a moderator between environment and anger control - in

The correlation of anger control-in with social relationships is moderated by the social network support. When the social network support is increasingly used by the patients, the relationship between anger control-in and social network is negative, which means that in case if the patients are using the social network the anger control-in increases and social network decreases.

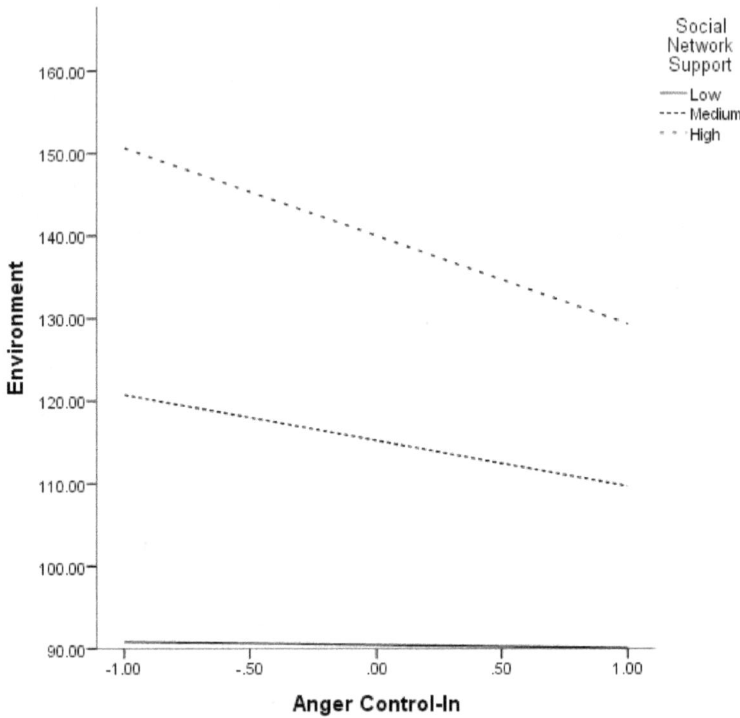

Figure 91. Social Network Support as a moderator between environment and anger control - in

The correlation of anger control-in with environment is moderated by the social network support. When the social network support is increasingly used by the patients, the relationship between anger control-in and environment is negative, which means that in case if the patients are using the social network the anger control-in increases and environment decreases.

Table 102

Moderating Effect of active focused coping strategies on Relationship of Anger Control-Out with Physical Health, Psychological Health, Social Relationships and Environment (n = 500)

Variables	Physical Health		Psychological health		Environment	
	$\triangle R^2$	β	$\triangle R^2$	β	$\triangle R^2$	β
Step 1						
Anger control-Out		2.21		-1.16		-2.55
Active focused coping		5.27		3.42		13.76***
Step 2	.00		.01		.01**	
Anger control-Out * Active focused coping		.01		.42		.89**
R^2	.074***		.25***		.54***	

***p < .001, ** p < .01, * p < .05.

Table 102 illustrates moderation analysis for active coping strategies in the relationship between anger control-out and quality of life (Physical functioning, Psychological functioning, Social relationships and Environment). Active focused coping strategies are acting as a moderator for the relationship of anger control-in with the environment. These added additional 5% of the variance is explained by this relationship of anger control-in and environment which is moderated by the active focused coping strategies. The moderating effect is further explained through mod graph.

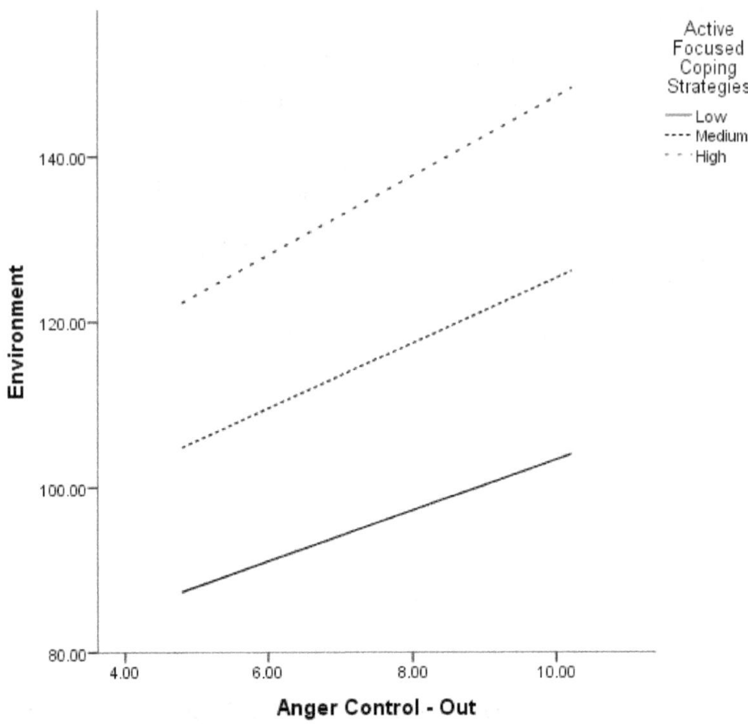

Figure 92. Active focused coping strategies as a moderator between environment and anger control - out

The correlation of anger control-out with environment is moderated by the active focused coping strategies. When the active focused coping strategies are increasingly used by the patients, the relationship between anger control-in and environment is positive, which means that in case if the patients are using the active focused coping strategies the anger control-out increases and environment also increases.

Table 103

Moderating Effect of avoidance focused coping strategies on Relationship of Anger Control-Out with Physical Health, Psychological Health and Environment (n = 500)

Variables	Physical Health		Psychological health		Environment	
	ΔR^2	β	ΔR^2	β	ΔR^2	β
Step 1						
Anger control-Out		4.13***		3.46***		2.14***
Avoidance focused coping strategies		9.35***		2.25***		12.21***
Step 2	.01**		.01		.00	
Anger control-Out * Avoidance focused coping strategies		1.89**		-.88		.71
R^2	.29***		.10***		.38***	

***$p < .001$, ** $p < .01$, * $p < .05$.

Table 103 illustrates moderation analysis for Avoidance focused coping strategies in the relationship between anger control-out and quality of life (Physical functioning, Psychological functioning and Environment). Avoidance focused coping strategies are acting as a moderator for the relationship of anger control-in with the physical health. It added additional 1% of the variance is explained by this relationship of anger control-out and physical health which is moderated by the avoidance focused coping strategies. The moderating effect is further explained through mod graph.

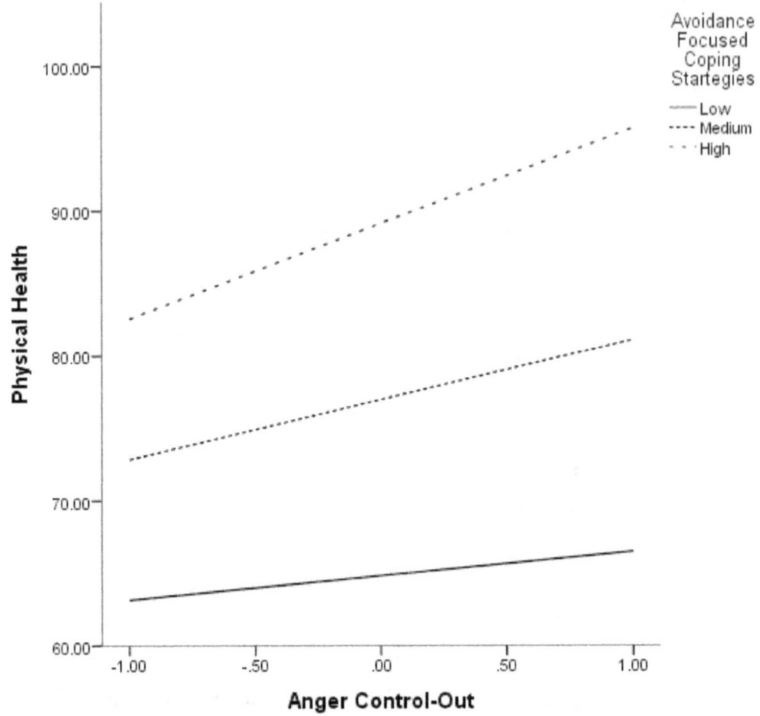

Figure 93. Avoidance focused coping strategies as a moderator between environment and anger control - out

The correlation of anger control-out with physical health is moderated by the avoidance focused coping strategies. When the avoidance focused coping strategies are increasingly used by the patients, the relationship between anger control-in and physical health is positive, which means that in case if the patients are using the avoidance focused coping strategies the anger control-out increases and physical also increases.

Table 104

Moderating Effect of Religious focused coping strategies on Relationship of Anger Control-Out with Physical Health, Psychological Health and Environment (n = 500)

Variables	Physical Health		Psychological health		Environment	
	ΔR^2	β	ΔR^2	β	ΔR^2	β
Step 1						
Anger control-Out		4.15**		3.67***		4.64***
Religious focused coping strategies		5.48***		1.46**		13.54**
Step 2	.01**		.00		.028***	
Anger control-Out * Religious focused coping strategies		3.10**		-.25		4.70***
R^2	.10***		.08***		.38***	

***$p < .001$, ** $p < .01$, * $p < .05$.

Table 104 illustrates moderation analysis for religious focused coping strategies in the relationship between anger control-out and quality of life (Physical functioning, Psychological functioning and Environment). Religious focused coping strategies are acting as a moderator for the relationship of anger control-in with the physical health. It added additional 1% of the variance is explained by this relationship of anger control-out and physical health which is moderated by the religious focused coping strategies. The moderating effect is further explained through mod graph.

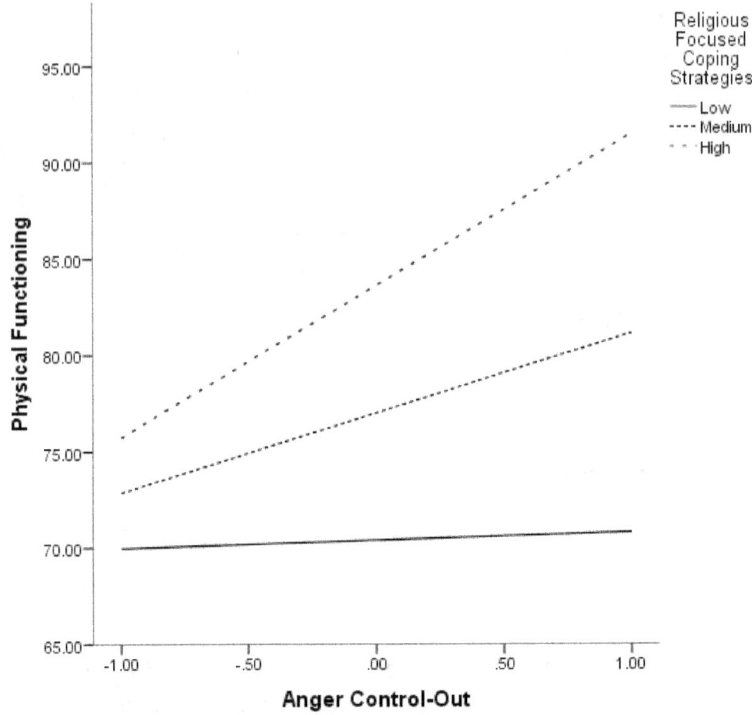

Figure 94. Religious focused coping strategies as a moderator between physical health and anger control - out

The correlation of anger control-out with physical health is moderated by the religious focused coping strategies. When the religious focused coping strategies are increasingly used by the patients, the relationship between anger control-in and physical health is positive, which means that in case if the patients are using the religious focused coping strategies the anger control-out increases and physical health or functioning also increases.

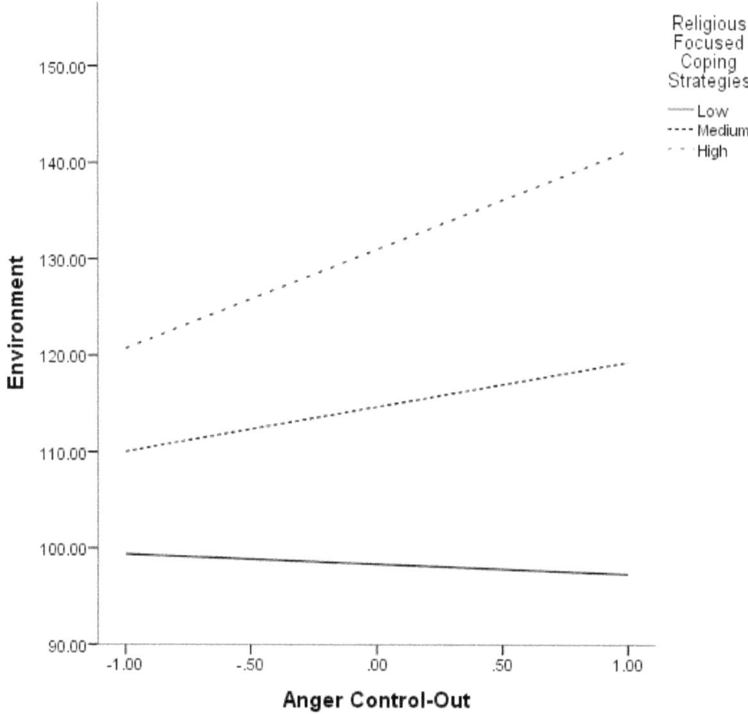

Figure 95. Religious focused coping strategies as a moderator between physical health and anger control - out

The correlation of anger control-out with environment is moderated by the religious focused coping strategies. When the religious focused coping strategies are increasingly used by the patients, the relationship between anger control-in and physical health is positive, which means that in case if the patients are using the religious focused coping strategies the anger control-out increases and environment also increases.

Table 105

Moderating Effect of Active distracting coping strategies on Relationship of Anger Control-Out with Physical Health, Psychological Health and Environment (n = 500)

Variables	Physical Health		Psychological health		Environment	
	$\triangle R^2$	β	$\triangle R^2$	β	$\triangle R^2$	β
Step 1						
Anger control-Out		4.13***		3.46***		5.14***
Active distracting coping strategies		9.35***		2.25***		12.21***
Step 2	.01**		.01		.00	
Anger control-Out * Active distracting coping strategies		1.89**		-.88		.71
R^2	.29***		.10***		.38***	

***$p < .001$, ** $p < .01$, * $p < .05$.

Table 105 illustrates moderation analysis for active distracting coping strategies in the relationship between anger control-out and quality of life (Physical functioning, Psychological functioning and Environment). Active distracting coping strategies are acting as a moderator for the relationship of anger control-in with the physical health. It added additional 1% of the variance is explained by this relationship of anger control-out and physical health which is moderated by the active distracting coping strategies. The moderating effect is further explained through mod graph.

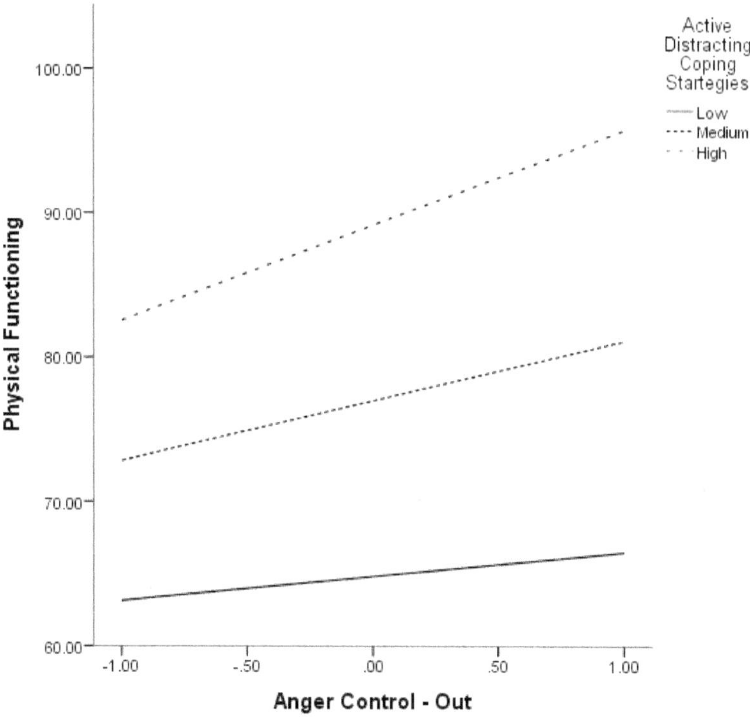

Figure 96. Active distracting coping strategies as a moderator between physical health and anger control - out

The correlation of anger control-out with physical health is moderated by the active distracting coping strategies. When the active distracting coping strategies are increasingly used by the patients, the relationship between anger control-in and physical health is positive, which means that in case if the patients are using the active distracting coping strategies the anger control-out increases and physical health or functioning also increases.

Table 106

Moderating Effect of Informational Support on Relationship of Anger Control-Out with Physical Health, Psychological Health and Environment (n = 500)

Variables	Physical Health		Psychological health		Environment	
	ΔR^2	β	ΔR^2	β	ΔR^2	β
Step 1						
Anger control-Out		4.66***		3.52***		5.63***
Informational Support		2.98*		1.07		10.04***
Step 2	.04***		.03**		.04***	
Anger control-Out * Informational Support		5.37***		2.46**		5.88***
R^2	.11***		.10***		.26***	

***$p < .001$, ** $p < .01$, * $p < .05$.

Table 106 illustrates moderation analysis for informational support in the relationship between anger control-out and quality of life (Physical functioning, Psychological functioning and Environment). Informational support is acting as a moderator for the relationship of anger control-in with the physical health. It added additional 4% of the variance is explained by this relationship of anger control-out and physical health which is moderated by the informational support. It also added additional 3% of the variance which is explained by the relationship of anger control-out and psychological functioning which is moderated by the informational support. Furthermore, it also added additional 4% of the variance which is explained by the relationship of anger control-out and environment which is moderated by the informational support. The moderating effect is further explained through mod graph.

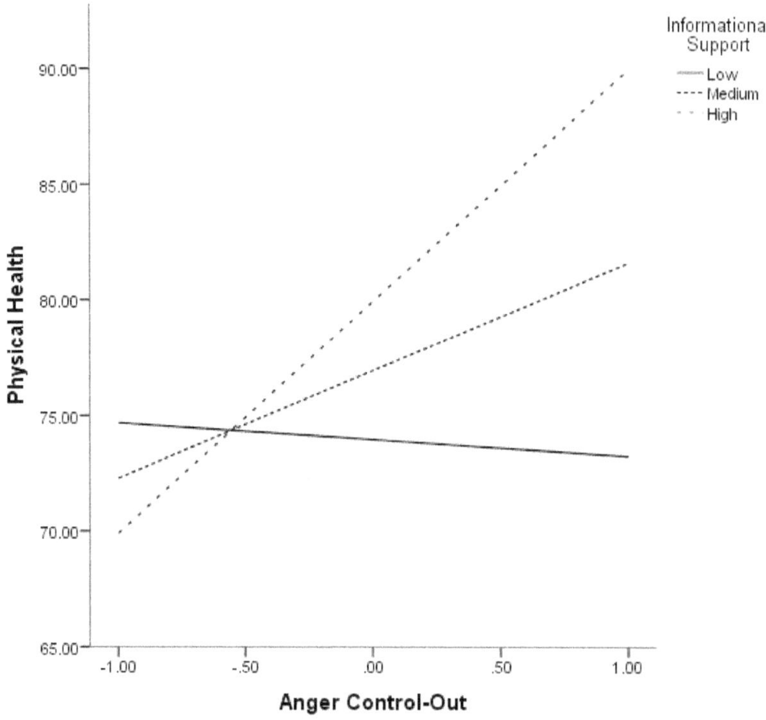

Figure 97. Informational support as a moderator between physical health and anger control - out

The correlation of anger control-out with physical health is moderated by the informational support. When the informational support is increasingly used by the patients, the relationship between anger control-out and physical is positive, which means that in case if the patients are using the informational support the anger control-out increases and physical health increase.

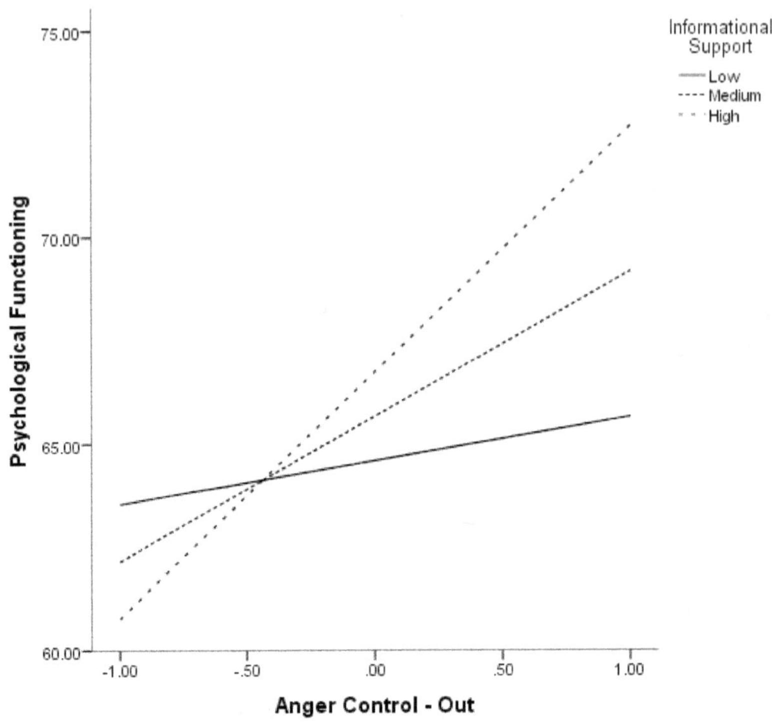

Figure 98. Informational support as a moderator between psychological functioning and anger control - out

The correlation of anger control-out with psychological functioning is moderated by the informational support. When the informational support is increasingly used by the patients, the relationship between anger control-out and psychological functioning is positive, which means that in case if the patients are using the informational support the anger control-out increases and psychological functioning increase.

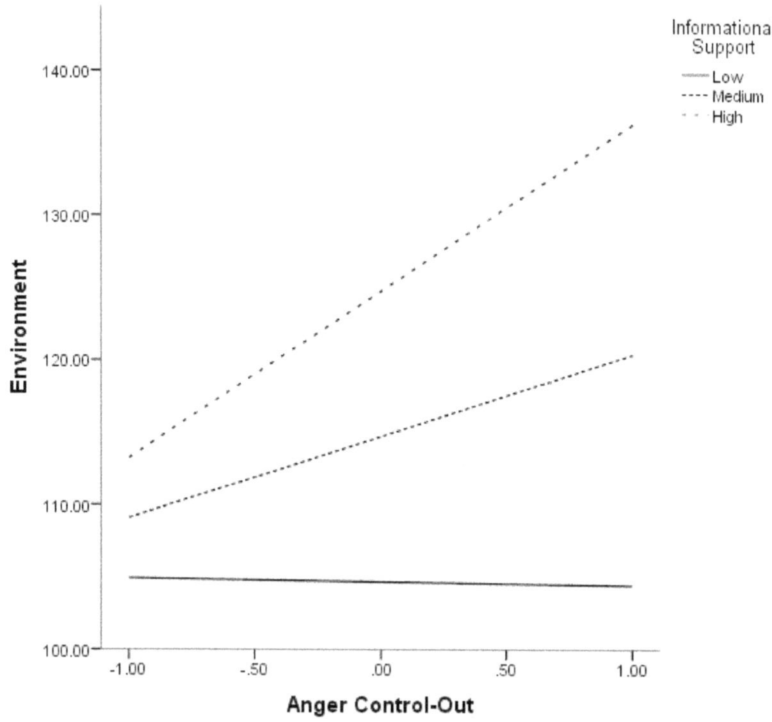

Figure 99. Informational support as a moderator between environment and anger control - out

The correlation of anger control-out with environment is moderated by the informational support. When the informational support is increasingly used by the patients, the relationship between anger control-out and environment is positive, which means that in case if the patients are using the informational support the anger control-out increases and environment increase.

Table 107

Moderating Effect of Tangible Support on Relationship of Anger Control-Out with Physical Health, Psychological Health and Environment (n = 500)

Variables	Physical Health		Psychological health		Environment	
	ΔR^2	β	ΔR^2	β	ΔR^2	β
Step 1						
Anger control-Out		5.03***		3.83***		6.36***
Tangible Support		4.63**		4.95***		13.89***
Step 2	.01*		.00		.05***	
Anger control-Out * Tangible Support		2.68*		.87		6.51***
R^2	.08***		.18***		.36***	

***$p < .001$, ** $p < .01$, * $p < .05$.

Table 107 illustrates moderation analysis for tangible support in the relationship between anger control-out and quality of life (Physical functioning, Psychological functioning and Environment). Tangible support is acting as a moderator for the relationship of anger control-in with the physical health. It added additional 1% of the variance is explained by this relationship of anger control-out and physical health which is moderated by the tangible support. Furthermore, it also added additional 5% of the variance which is explained by the relationship of anger control-out and environment which is moderated by the tangible support. The moderating effect is further explained through mod graph.

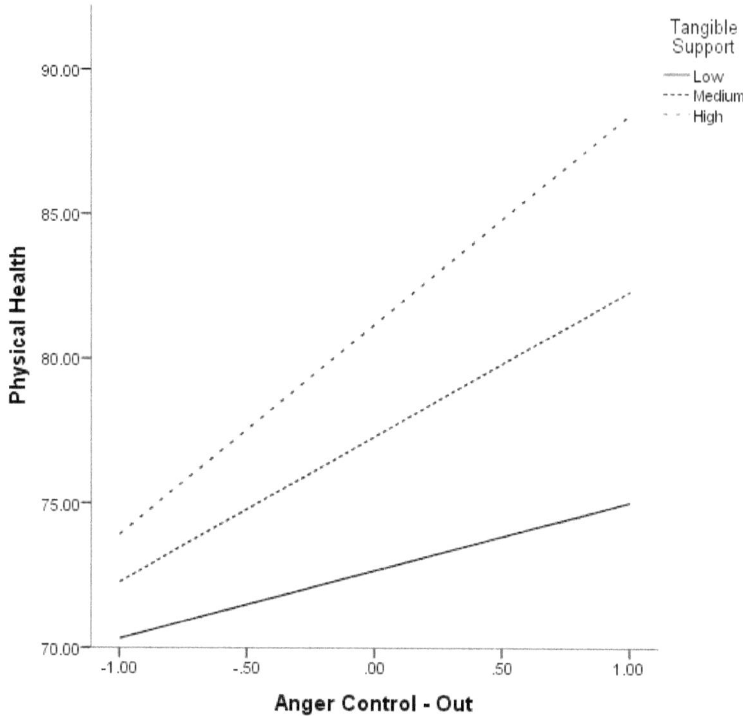

Figure 100. Tangible support as a moderator between physical health and anger control - out

The correlation of anger control-out with physical health is moderated by the tangible support. When the tangible support is increasingly used by the patients, the relationship between anger control-out and physical is positive, which means that in case if the patients are using the tangible support the anger control-out increases and physical health increase.

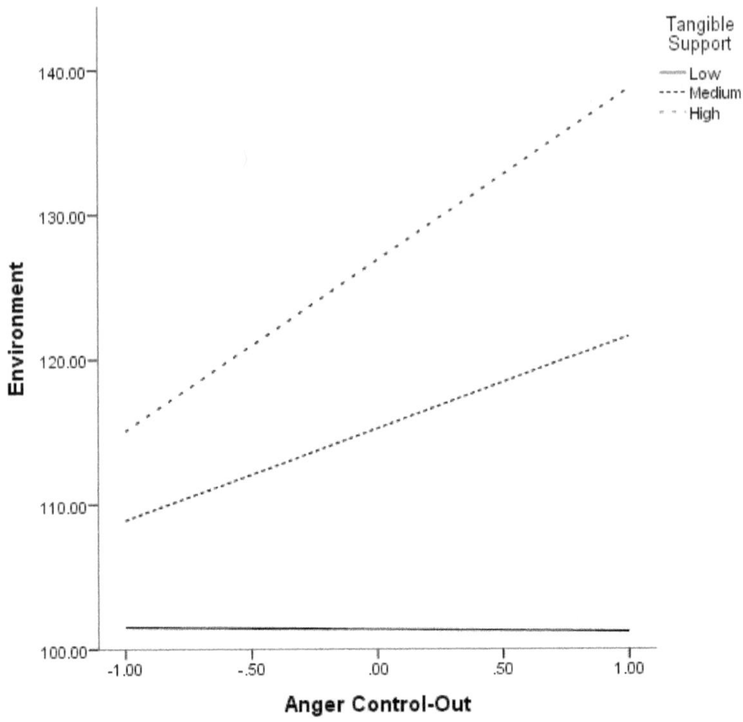

Figure 101. Tangible support as a moderator between environment and anger control - out

The correlation of anger control-out with environment is moderated by the tangible support. When the tangible support is increasingly used by the patients, the relationship between anger control-out and environment is positive, which means that in case if the patients are using the tangible support the anger control-out increases and environment increase.

Table 108

Moderating Effect of Emotional Support on Relationship of Anger Control-Out with Physical Health, Psychological Health and Environment (n = 500)

Variables	Physical Health		Psychological health		Environment	
	ΔR^2	β	ΔR^2	β	ΔR^2	β
Step 1						
Anger control-Out		4.87***		3.43***		5.69***
Emotional Support		8.71***		4.66***		18.55***
Step 2	.31		.02*		.00	
Anger control-Out * Emotional Support		-1.16		1.89*		1.46
R^2	.13***		.23***		.53***	

***$p < .001$, ** $p < .01$, * $p < .05$.

Table 108 illustrates moderation analysis for emotional support in the relationship between anger control-out and quality of life (Physical functioning, Psychological functioning and Environment). Emotional support is acting as a moderator for the relationship of anger control-in with the psychological health. It added additional 2% of the variance is explained by this relationship of anger control-out and psychological functioning which is moderated by the tangible support. The moderating effect is further explained through mod graph.

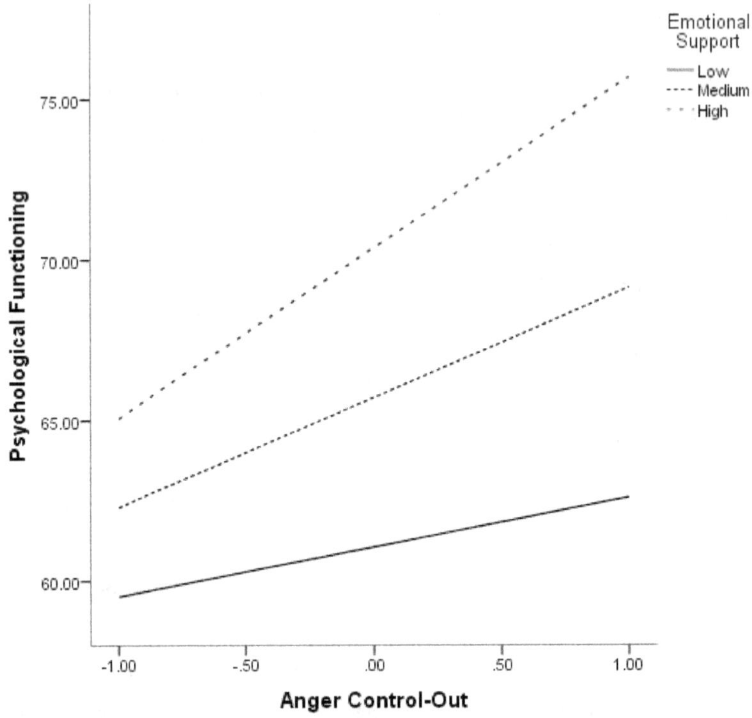

Figure 102. Emotional support as a moderator between psychological functioning and anger control - out

The association between the anger control-out and psychological functioning is moderated by the emotional support. When the emotional support is increasingly used by the patients, the relationship between anger control-out and psychological functioning is positive, which means that in case if the patients are using the emotional support the anger control-out increases and psychological functioning increase.

Table 109

Moderating Effect of Esteem Support on Relationship of Anger Control-Out with Physical Health, Psychological Health and Environment (n = 500)

Variables	Physical Health		Psychological health		Environment	
	$\triangle R^2$	β	$\triangle R^2$	β	$\triangle R^2$	β
Step 1						
Anger control-Out		5.52***		3.96***		7.38***
Esteem Support		7.15***		5.02***		17.95***
Step 2	.00		.01*		.01*	
Anger control-Out * Esteem Support		-.53		1.39*		2.61*
R^2	.10***		.22***		.52***	

$***p < .001, ** p < .01, * p < .05.$

Table 109 illustrates moderation analysis for esteem support in the relationship between anger control-out and quality of life (Physical functioning, Psychological functioning and Environment). Esteem support is acting as a moderator for the relationship of anger control-in with the psychological health. It added additional 1% of the variance is explained by this relationship of anger control-out and psychological functioning which is moderated by the esteem support. Furthermore, it added additional 1% of the variance is explained by this relationship of anger control-out and environment which is moderated by the esteem support. The moderating effect is further explained through mod graph.

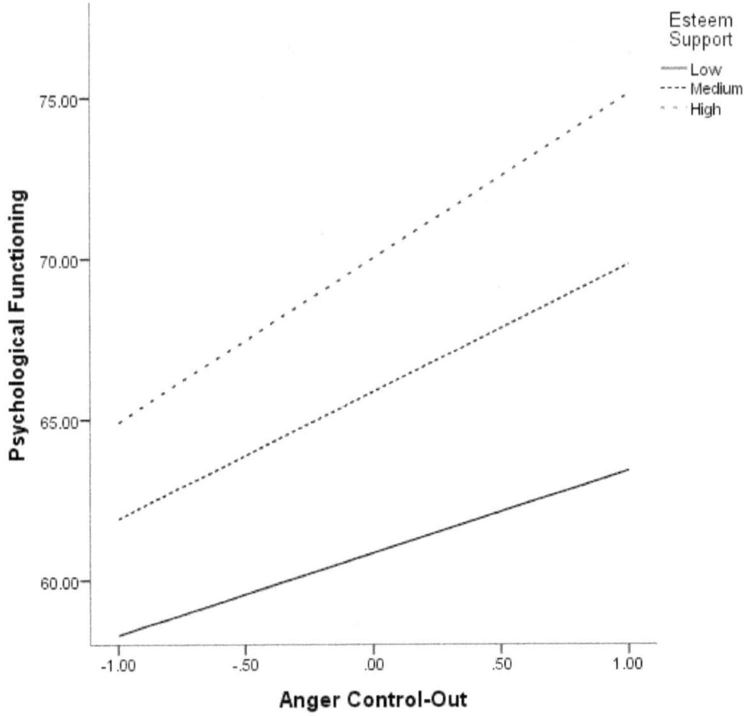

Figure 103. Esteem support as a moderator between psychological functioning and anger control - out

The correlation of anger control-out with psychological functioning is moderated by the esteem support. When the esteem support is increasingly used by the patients, the relationship between anger control-out and psychological functioning is positive, which means that in case if the patients are using the esteem support the anger control-out increases and psychological functioning increase.

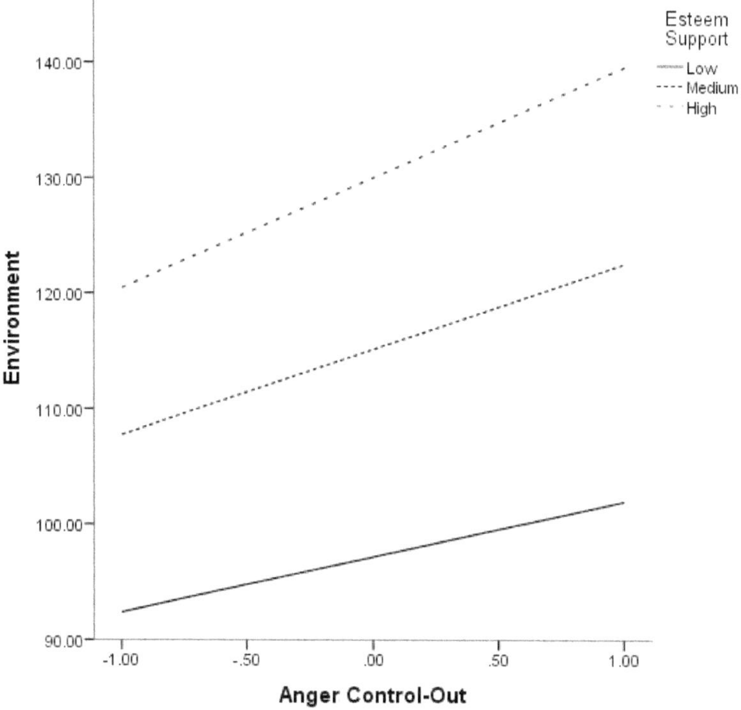

Figure 104. Esteem support as a moderator between environment and anger control - out

The correlation of anger control-out with environment is moderated by the esteem support. When the esteem support is increasingly used by the patients, the relationship between anger control-out and environment is positive, which means that in case if the patients are using the esteem support the anger control-out increases and environment increase.

Table 110

Moderating Effect of Social Networking Support on Relationship of Anger Control-Out with Physical Health, Psychological Health and Environment (n = 500)

Variables	Physical Health		Psychological health		Environment	
	ΔR^2	β	ΔR^2	β	ΔR^2	β
Step 1						
Anger control-Out		2.37**		1.97**		1.59*
Social Networking Support		13.511***		8.36***		22.72***
Step 2	.00		.01*		.03***	
Anger control-Out * Social Networking Support		-1.41		1.29*		4.40***
R^2	.28***		.39***		.73***	

***$p < .001$, ** $p < .01$, * $p < .05$.

Table 110 illustrates moderation analysis for social networking support in the relationship between anger control-out and quality of life (Physical functioning, Psychological functioning and Environment). Social Networking support is acting as a moderator for the relationship of anger control-in with the psychological health. It added additional 1% of the variance is explained by this relationship of anger control-out and psychological functioning which is moderated by the social networking support. Furthermore, it added additional 3% of the variance is explained by this relationship of anger control-out and environment which is moderated by the social networking support. The moderating effect is further explained through mod graph.

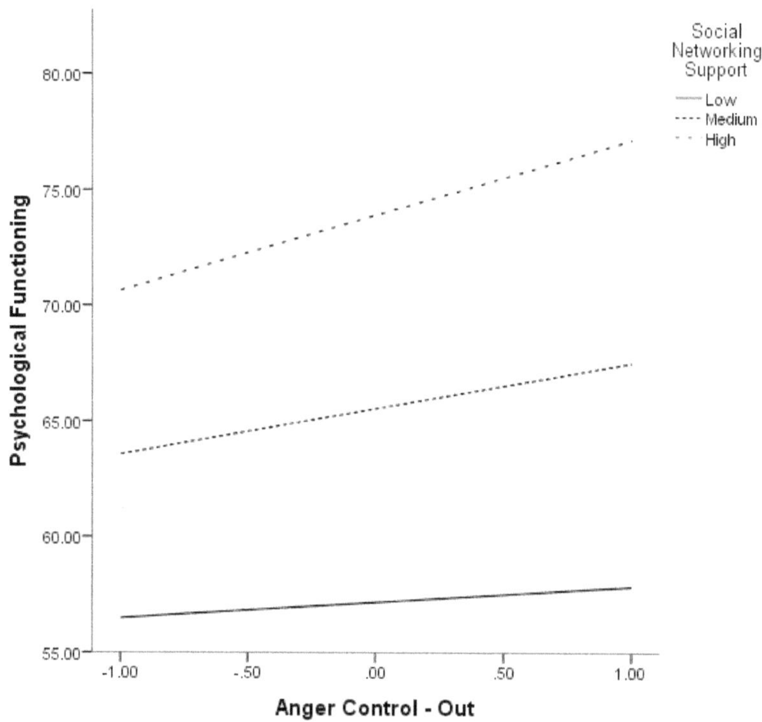

Figure 105.   Social Networking support as a moderator between psychological functioning and anger control - out

The correlation of anger control-out with psychological functioning is moderated by the social networking support. When the social networking support is increasingly used by the patients, the relationship between anger control-out and psychological functioning is positive, which means that in case if the patients are using the social networking support the anger control-out increases and psychological functioning increase.

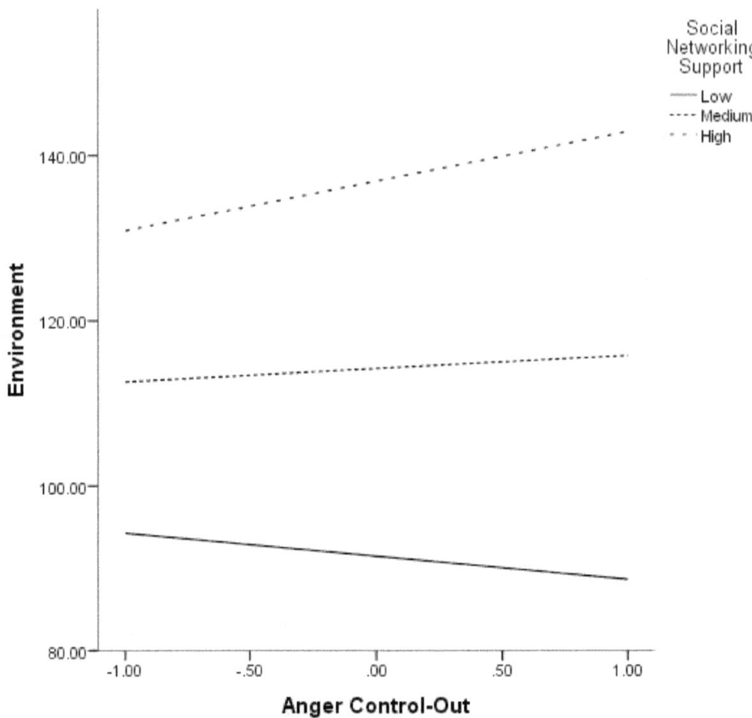

Figure 106. Social Networking support as a moderator between environment and anger control - out

The correlation of anger control-out with environment is moderated by the social networking support. When the social networking support is increasingly used by the patients, the relationship between anger control-out and environment is positive, which means that in case if the patients are using the social networking support the anger control-out increases and environment increase.

Multivariate and Univariate Analysis

Table 111

Multivariate and univariate Analysis of demographic Variables of the present Study (N=500)

Variables	MANOVA F	ANOVA F																								
		1	2	3	4	5	6	7	8	9	10	11	12	13	14	15	16	17	18	19	20	21	22	23	24
E X M	1.67***	3.96**	1.06	1.67	2.52	.84	.15	.59	.47	.54	.20	.56	1.76	2.12	.92	.35	.93	.70	.47	5.29***	4.37**	3.51*	4.56**	3.77*	5.48**
E X A	1.41**	3.05*	1.00	.43	.24	1.24	1.38	1.37	.38	2.97*	.85	4.29*	4.41*	6.94***	3.79**	1.06	4.31**	4.48**	1.36	10.24***	7.57***	2.48	9.18***	6.94***	4.05**

Note. *F* ratios are Wilk's approximation of *F*. ANOVA = univariate analysis of variance; MANOVA=multivariate analysis of variance;; A=age, O= occupation; M= marital status; 1= Depression, 2 = State Anger, 3= Anger Control-In, 4=Anger Control-Out, 5=Active focused Coping strategies, 6=Active Distractive Focused Coping Strategies, 7= Avoidance Focused Coping Strategies. 8= Religious Focused Coping Strategies, 9= Informational Support, 10= Tangible Support, 11= Emotional Support, 12= Esteem Support, 13 = Social Network Support, 14 = Physical Functioning, 15 = Psychological Functioning, 16 = Social Relationships. 17 = Environment, 18 = Perceived Quality. 19 = Environmental Mastery, 20 = Self-Acceptance. 21 = Positive relations with others. 22= autonomy, 23 = Purpose In Life, 24 = Personal Growth.

p < .05.**p* <..001. ***p* <.0001.

Table 111 presents findings of multivariate analyses for assessing the influence of demographics on variables of the present study. Among all the factors, the only education had a significant multivariate F whereas all other factors (including disease, disease duration, gender, marital status and age) were non-significant in relation to the combination of variables of the present study. The significant multivariate main effect of education and marital status, education with age was followed by univariate analyses of variance, which have shown significant differences in depression, informational support, social network support, environmental mastery, self-acceptance, autonomy, purpose in life and personal growth.

Table 112

Means, standard deviation and t-values of gender wise differences on ascip, beck depression inventory, coping strategies questionnaire, social support questionnaire, psychological well-being questionnaire and quality of life questionnaire of chronically patients and diabetic patients (n=500).

	Male (n = 131)		Female (n = 369)		t	p	95% CI		Cohen's d
	M	SD	M	SD			LL	UL	
Depression	15.63	13.61	15.27	13.92	.26	.54	-2.41	3.13	0.03
State anger	13.50	5.70	12.72	4.70	1.54	.01	-.21	1.78	0.15
Anger control-in	19.63	7.21	20.91	6.68	1.84	.05	-2.64	.09	0.18
Anger control-out	7.36	2.79	7.55	2.68	.70	.53	-.74	.35	0.07
Active focused coping strategies	7.39	1.02	7.24	.95	1.50	.36	-.05	.34	0.15
Active distracting coping	6.70	1.35	6.51	1.28	1.48	.19	-.06	.46	0.14
Avoidance focused coping	6.40	.61	6.33	.69	1.09	.11	-.60	.21	0.11
Religious focused coping	7.23	1.11	6.84	1.22	3.21	.09	.15	.63	0.33
Informational support	18.54	4.30	19.15	3.58	1.59	.01	-1.37	.14	0.15
Tangible support	16.42	4.60	17.18	3.17	2.08	.00	-1.48	-.04	0.19
Emotional support	54.23	5.59	54.28	5.57	.10	.30	-1.12	1.02	0.01
Esteem support	40.07	5.59	39.68	5.09	.75	.51	-.63	1.40	0.07

Continued...

| | Male | | Female | | t | p | 95% CI | | Cohen's |
	(*n* = 131)		(*n* = 369)						*d*
	M	*SD*	*M*	*SD*			*LL*	*UL*	
Social network support	41.43	5.25	40.96	5.42	.86	.36	-.61	1.54	0.09
Physical functioning	78.90	27.60	76.60	26.15	.85	.31	-2.10	7.61	0.09
Psychological functioning	64.18	16.70	66.35	14.08	1.44	.05	-5.13	.79	0.14
Social relationships	44.34	15.25	39.89	14.69	2.95	.25	1.79	7.42	0.30
Environment	119.39	28.77	113.43	28.01	2.08	.96	.32	11.60	0.21
Perceived quality of life	13.62	5.52	13.88	5.28	.47	.30	-1.33	.811	0.05
Environmental mastery	27.38	15.29	33.01	13.46	3.96	.000	-8.41	-2.84	0.39
Self – acceptance	30.78	11.79	34.41	11.29	3.13	.44	-5.92	-1.35	0.31
Positive relations with others	29.92	11.93	34.79	10.50	4.40	.003	-7.06	-2.70	0.43
Autonomy	36.40	11.07	33.16	11.06	2.89	.49	1.04	5.45	0.29
Purpose in life	28.27	10.59	32.06	10.49	3.54	.62	-5.89	-1.69	0.36
Personal growth	26.73	11.31	31.88	10.31	4.78	.02	-7.26	-2.83	0.48

Results in the table 112 indicates that the tangible support, environmental mastery, positive relations with others and personal growth is significantly high among female patients as compared to males.

Table 113

Means, Standard deviation and t-values of Family System Wise Differences on ASCIP, Beck Depression Inventory, Coping Strategies Questionnaire, Social Support Questionnaire, Psychological Well-Being Questionnaire and Quality of Life Questionnaire of Chronically Patients and Diabetic Patients (n=500)

	Nuclear (*n* =286)		Joint(*n* = 214)		*t*	*p*	95% CI		Cohen's d
	M	*SD*	*M*	*SD*			*LL*	*UL*	
Depression	16.74	15.36	13.51	11.23	2.60	.000	.80	5.68	0.24
State anger	12.71	4.72	13.21	5.32	1.11	.07	-1.38	.38	0.10
Anger control-in	20.23	6.87	21.03	6.79	1.29	.56	-2.01	.42	0.12
Anger control-out	7.59	2.82	7.38	2.56	.85	.01	-.27	.69	0.08
Active focused coping strategies	7.28	.97	7.27	.97	.11	.67	-.16	.18	0.01
Active distracting coping	6.57	1.33	6.54	1.27	.24	.31	-.20	.26	0.02
Avoidance focused coping	6.34	.64	6.36	.71	.45	.57	-.15	.09	0.03
Religious focused coping	6.98	1.20	6.91	1.22	.64	.94	-.14	.29	0.06
Informational support	18.83	3.94	19.21	3.56	1.11	.07	-1.05	.29	0.10
Tangible support	16.76	3.92	17.27	3.13	1.56	.01	-1.15	.13	0.14
Emotional support	54.27	5.57	54.26	5.05	.02	.26	-.94	.96	0.002
Esteem support	39.74	5.17	39.84	4.99	.20	.51	-.10	.81	0.02
Social network support	41.14	5.44	41.00	5.29	.28	.56	-.82	1.09	0.03
Physical functioning	78.49	26.75	75.48	26.19	1.26	.32	-1.70	7.72	0.11
Psychological functioning	65.41	15.60	66.28	13.74	.65	.24	-3.45	1.77	0.06
Social relationships	41.99	14.76	39.79	15.15	1.62	.89	-.46	4.84	0.15
Environment	115.78	28.99	113.94	27.39	.72	.15	-3.20	6.86	0.07

Continued...

	Nuclear (n = 286)		Joint(n = 214)		t	p	95% CI		Cohen's d
	M	SD	M	SD			LL	UL	
Perceived quality of life	13.66	5.38	14.00	5.30	.70	.49	-1.28	.61	0.06
Environmental mastery	29.47	14.39	34.29	13.40	3.82	.000	-7.30	-2.34	0.35
Self – acceptance	31.89	11.62	35.57	11.09	3.57	.25	-5.70	-1.65	0.32
Positive relations with others	32.02	11.39	35.51	10.38	3.52	.000	-5.44	-1.55	0.32
Autonomy	35.20	11.39	32.43	10.81	2.78	.80	.81	4.73	0.25
Purpose in life	29.53	10.85	33.12	10.01	3.78	.001	-5.45	-1.72	0.34
Personal growth	29.09	10.90	32.44	10.41	3.47	.002	-5.25	-1.45	0.31

Results in Table 113 indicate that the depression is significantly high among those patients who are from nuclear family system whereas environmental mastery, positive relations with others and personal growth is high among those patients who are from joint family system.

Chapter VI

DISCUSSION

The present study was conducted to explore the psychological issues, risk and protective factors of patients (chronically ill). Furthermore, it also aimed to explore the risk and protective factors with particular reference to psychological well-being and quality of life of patients. The study was conducted in two parts. Part- I of the study comprised of three phases. Phase I dealt with the finalization of study variables through focus groups and interviews, Phase–II comprised of the Instrument development and Phase–III dealt with the establishment of the psychometric properties of the instruments. Part–II is comprised of the main study that aimed to test the study hypotheses particularly.

In Part II, the focus was to identify psychological issues most commonly reported by chronically ill patients. As discussed in previous part of present study, these psychological issues were labeled as depression and anger, the prevalence of depression and anger highlighted the significance of these issues. Further, the predictive relationship of depression and anger for quality of life and psychological well-being of chronically ill patients (cardiac, cancer and diabetics) strengthen the need to focus on these issues. The study also aimed to find out the moderating role of risk and protective factors (social support and coping) in relationship of psychological issues and quality of life and psychological well-being.

Prevalence of Psychological Issues

The findings depicted that the prevalence of depression and anger is significantly high among cardiac patients as compared to cancer and diabetes patients. Existing literature support the notion that chronically ill patients do report symptoms of depression and anger (Davidson & Mostofsy, 2010; Ilic & Apostolovic, 2002). Literature provides the same picture about the cardiac patients and revealed that approximately 20% of the patients with coronary heart disease (CHD) have been suffering from major depression and 20% have mild depression at any given point of time during the course of their illness (Carney & Freedland, 2008). Results also indicate that the patients of diabetes and cancer also suffer from mild to moderate level of depression. Depression is commonly reported among diabetic (Anderston, Freedland, Clouse & Lustman, 2001; Lewko & Misiak, 2014; Mir, Mir, Malik, Quratulain, & Shehzadi, 2015) and cancer patients (Hadi, Asadollahi, & Talei, 2009; Pasquini & Biondi, 2007).

In a country like Pakistan people are hardly earning their bread and butter, in that state if they suffer from the chronic illness that is actually adding up to their misery. As it has been explained in 1939 by Dollard et al in Frustration-agreesion hypothesis that one may experiences frustration because of the blockage of one's goal directed behavior, the person may suffer first from frustration and then from aggression (DiGiuseppe, & Tafrate, 2007). Sometimes the people who are suffering from chronic illness suffer from the feeling of hopelessness and then afterwards suffer from helplessness which leads to the phenomenon of learned helplessness. These feelings mostly left the person with nothing not even with hope (Lubkin & Larsen, 2006). The repitive failtures of an individual makes him learn that he is a complete failure no matter whatever the situation is going to be, he will only endup with failure in every area of his life (Dalal, 2015). With the realization of the fact that one is having a chronic illness, is related with the significant impact in one's life. Individuals may suffer or experience the feelings of depression, helplessness, apathy and hopelessness. They feel rejected and dejected (Falvo & Holland, 2017).

Cancer is the second leading cause of death in U.S. The age adjusted cancer death rates are increasing in the US population (Bal & Foerster, 1991). There are many types of cancers but the most common include carcinoma, sarcoma, lymphoma and leukemia. There are many other types of cancer, depending on the body part which get affected by the cancer. In Pakistan the registered cases are very few. A big dilemma is that most of the patients die of some chronic illnesses but that never get diagnosed. Karachi Cancer Registry (KCR) was developed for documentation and registration of cancer. It is providing the prevalence of cancer in the country (Bano et al., 2013). There are many cases which never get diagnosed as they don't have access to the medical facilities that's why their diseases mostly go undiagnosed. Cancer is more closely tied with the life style then to genetics (Lichtenstein et al., 2000). The diagnosis of having cancer is shocking, heartbreaking and earth shaking for the patients. Facing a cancer is a tragic event of patient's life which may lead to significant psychological distress and appearance of the psychiatric symptoms, such as sleep difficulty, excessive worries regarding survival and depressive mood. These symptoms are often associated with lower quality of life and well-being (Bornbaum et al., 2012; Oh, Seo, Jeong, & Seo, 2013). Lots of problems are linked with the diagnosis of the chronic illness (Heather, Susan, Deanna, & Barbara, 2006; National Cancer Registry, 2003; Senescus, 1963). Depression, anxiety disorders, adjustment disorder, and sickness states are common among cancer patients (Gregurek et al., 2010; Taylor, 2006).

Diagnoses of the disease are shocking and distressing event for the patients and the treatment is something which is above all. It is adding fear and tension in the life of the patients. During treatment many patients develop many psychological issues. All cancer patients experience some level of distress linked with the cancer and its treatment (all stages) of the disease (Derogatis, Morrow, & Fetting, 1983).

Just like cancer, diabetes is also a chronic illness and always adding up to the tensions of the patients. In the country like Pakistan where there is no well established information system related to the course of treatment of the patients. Health professionals working with diabetes patients often fail to identify psychological problems and disorders. Approximately two out of three patients with serious psychological problems remain undiagnosed (Hermanns, Kulzer, Krichbaum, Kubiak, & Haak, 2006; Pouwer, Beekman, Lubach, & Snoek, 2006).

As per according to one report the cases of diabetes are increasing day and night, many have impaired glucose level of tolerace which is adding up to the problems, male and female prevelance ratio varies from rural to urban areas but prevlance rate is increasing irrespective of geographical regions (Aziz, Noorulain, Zaidi, Hossain, & Siddiqui, 2009). These statistics clearly indicates the high prevalence of diabetes, issues and problems always accompany the disease. The physical problems associated with diabetes are excessive thirst, polyuria, weight loss, loss of energy etc. and patients are unable to carry out their daily life activities so it is adding up to their tensions that's why slowly gradually they develop psychological disorders. It is commonly reported that many patients who are already suffering from chronic illness get diagnosed with depression, hopelessness, mood problems, sometime they have a strong desire to commit suicide and also suffer from other psychological problems (Turner & Brian, 2000).

In the present study the mild, moderate and severe level of state anger, anger control-in and anger control – out was determined with below 20th, between 20th to 80th and severe with above 80th percentile respectively. It has been observed that previous literature (Crawford, Cayley, Lovibond, Wilson & Hartley, 2011; Shahid, Wilkinson, Marcu & Shapiro, 2012) also indicates that categories can be generated on the basis of percentile ranks. The results of the present study further revealed that the cardiac patients have significantly high level of state anger as compared to cancer and diabetes patients. They suffer from severe level of anger. Literature highlights that the hostility is commonly reported among the cardiac patients (Ilic & Apostolovic, 2002). Moderate to severe level of state anger is found in all patients (cardiac, diabetics and cardiac) but large number of cardiac patients has state anger as compared to the diabetic and cancer patients. All patients suffer from anger and the justification could be given with reference to the FGDs and interviews conducted in the Phase – I of the Part – I of the present study, it was commonly reported by the patients that they are sick and tired of being in the hospital and it's very frustrating for them to be on bed and doing nothing. They feel like they have lost their life interest and activities so they sometimes experience anger. Patients said that they have lost interest in their lives and preferring dying over that type of life. They don't want to be dependent but disease has made them dependent that's they develop psychological issues. It was revealed from the comments and discussions of the patients and caregivers that the patients in Pakistan are being influenced by many challenges including physical dependency, financial insecurities, living issues, uncertainty in treatment and its outcome, no awareness about stage of their disease or illness and also the course of treatment.

Results of the present study revealed that the cancer patients suffer from depression which ranges from mild to moderate level of depression. It also reveals that the cancer patients also suffer from moderate to severe level of anger. The findings are consistent with the findings of the research in which it was figured out that the patients commonly suffer from the negative mood along with the low energy, poor concentration, loss of interests, memory disturbances, sleep difficulty and hopelessness are the common complaints of the patients which are direct indication of major Depressive Disorder. Many patients also show the symptoms of anger, irritability and hostility (Biondi, Picardi, Pasquini, Gaetano, & Pancheri, 2005; Pasquini, Picardi, Biondi, Gaetano, & Morosini, 2004).

Relationship of Psychological issues with Psychological Well-Being and Quality of Life

Current study results highlighted that there is a significant negative relationship of depression with psychological well-being (environmental mastery, self-acceptance, purpose in life, personal growth, autonomy and positive relations with others) and quality of life (psychological functioning and environment) among chronically ill patients. State anger is also negatively associated with quality of life (psychological functioning, social relationships and environment) among chronically ill patients. Anger control-in is also having a significant negative relationship with psychological well-being (environmental mastery, purpose in life, personal growth and positive relations with others) and quality of life (psychological functioning, social relationships and environment) among chronically ill patients. Whereas Anger Control – out is positively associated with quality of life (physical functioning, psychological functioning and environment) among chronically ill patients.

It is evident that chronically ill patients having psychological problems have worst quality of life and psychological well-being. It has been established in the literature that there is a bidirectional relationship between depression and chronic medical conditions. The undesirable health risk behaviors and biological changes and problematic conditions are associated with the depression. This association increases the risk behaviors and biological changes and complications. Depression may worsen the course of the medical condition of the patients suffering from diabetes and cardiac diseases (Katon, 2011). Pattern (2001) established in a large Canadian community based study that there was an increased risk of development of depression among chronically ill patients as compared to those who are without it (Pattern, 2001).

The high level of depression is going to have a devastating impact on the quality of life of CHD patients (Carney & Freedland, 2008). People with cardiovascular conditions or diabetes had higher risk of reporting poor health related quality of life outcomes than those with other chronic conditions (Chen, Baumgardner & Rice, 2011). There is a significant negative relationship between depression and psychological well-being among diabetic patients (Ramkisson, Pillay, & Sartorious, 2016). Current study results have supported the literature guidelines and it was found that if psychological issues increase the quality of life and psychological well-being decreases, hence hypotheses one and two are fully supported.

Predictive Role of Psychological Issues for Well-Being and Quality of Life

The multiple regression analysis revealed that psychological issues (depression and anger) are significantly predicting the well-being (psychological) and quality of life of chronically ill patients. Quality of life of chronically ill patient is judged by the disruption in sleep, appetite gets affected and the daily functioning gets affected. In the latter stages and at more chronic stage quality of life is associated with the fact that whether the individual is able to perform independently the daily routine activities like eating, bathing, dressing etc. inability to perform these daily activities independently adversely affect the psychological condition of the person (Ghosh, 2015). Universally, quality of life is assessed, based on certain components like performing different daily physical activities, emotionally one is sound, interpersonal relationships, personal control, energy level, social functioning, personal and intellectual growth etc. (Power, Harper & Bullinger, 1999).

Present study results revealed that depression significantly predicts the psychological well-being (environmental mastery, autonomy, personal growth, positive relations with other, purpose in life, self-acceptance) and quality of life (social relationships). Results indicate that as the depression increases the psychological well-being and quality of life decreases, in case the person is suffering from depression then his or her quality of life and psychological well-being can easily be predicted. It has been highlighted in the literature that the chronically ill patients have diminished or deteriorated quality of life and their wellbeing also get effected because of depression (Casper, 2015) State anger significantly predicts psychological well-being (environmental mastery, personal growth) and quality of life (physical functioning, social relationships and environment). State anger according to literature (Etzler, Rohrmann, & Brandnt, 2014) is basically linked with the state or situation in which person is experiencing or witnessing something. State affects the mind set and behavior of the person. Anger control – in significantly predicts psychological well-being (autonomy, positive relations with other, self-acceptance) quality of life (psychological functioning, social relationships and environment). Anger control – out significantly predicts quality of life (psychological functioning and environment), hence hypothesis two is supported by this finding. Literature also revealed that depression and anger significantly predicts the quality of life among chronically ill patients (Abu-Helalah, Al-Hanaqta, Alshraideh, Abdulbaqi, & Hijazeen, 2014; Wu, 2014).

Moderating Role of Social Support and Coping Strategies

Results revealed that Social support (tangible support, social network support) was explored as moderator in relationship between depression and psychological well- being (self -acceptance, positive relationship with other and autonomy), whereas esteem support acted as moderator between relationship of state anger and psychological well -being (environmental mastery, personal growth). Avoidance focused coping strategies and Active distracting coping strategies were acting as a moderator for the relationship of depression with psychological well-being (environmental mastery, self-acceptance, positive relations, purpose in life, autonomy, social relationships and personal growth). The result indicates that when the patients increasingly use the avoidance focused coping, and active distractive coping strategies, the depression increases and psychological wellbeing (environmental mastery, self-acceptance, positive relations with others, purpose in life, autonomy, social relationships and personal growth) decreases. Another surprising finding is that the patients those who are using active focused they also sometimes get frustrated and in a result their depression gets aggravated. Sometimes patients get tired with the even doing something for the betterment of their health but still they find these efforts going into vein as they are not giving them anything in return. With all efforts their health is not improving which is clearly mentioned by patients in their interviews which they have given in the Part –I of Phase – I of the present study. Religious focused coping strategies were acting as a moderator in the relationship of depression with environmental mastery, positive relations and personal growth. Religious focused support is sometimes proving as a great help in improving the psychological well-being of the patients but sometimes not. As reported in the literature that the religiousity is playing the role of moderator in correlation of chronic medical condition and the psychological well-being of the patients (Abolfathi Momtaz, Hamid, Ibrahim, Yahaya, & Abdullah, 2012).

Tangible support, Social Network Support, esteem support and social network support were acting as a moderator for the relationship of depression with psychological well-being (self-acceptance, autonomy, environmental mastery, positive relations with others and personal growth). As indicated by the literature that there are some risk factors such as duration of illness or disease, age, low social support, individual factors like defensive coping they may increase the likelihood of negative buffering effects of psychological issues on individual's mental and psychological functioning (Haung, 2009), whereas, some protective factors (i.e., social support and coping strategies) may intervene to save the individuals from these negative influences (i.e., depression, hopelessness, mood problems, sometime they commit suicide etc.) (Turner & Brian, 2000). Informational support, emotional support, esteem support, and social networking support were acting as a moderator for the relationship of state anger with environmental mastery and personal growth. In case if excessive social support (informational, emotional, esteem and social networking support is available to the patients, again it effects the patients adversely but if moderate level of social support will get available to them it will help in dealing with disease effectively. Social support has been identified as an important factor alleviating psychological issues (depression) in cancer patients (Bailey et al., 2005). Social support has positive effect on physical and psychological well-being of people suffering from chronic illness such as cancer (Helgeson & Cohen, 1996). Social support affects the well-being of the patients (Swindells et al., 1999). It has also been reported that social support plays a moderating role in relationship between depressive symptoms and quality of life of cancer patients (Huang & Hsu, 2013). Informational support acted as a moderator in the relationship of anger control-In with positive relations with others. Emotional support was acting as a moderator for the relationship of anger control-In with self-acceptance and positive relations with others. Esteem support also acted as a moderator in the relationship of anger control-In with self-acceptance. Emotional support was also acted as a moderator for the relationship of anger control-in with the psychological health. Esteem support is acting as a moderator in the relationship of anger control-in with the psychological health. Social Networking support is acting as a moderator in the relationship of anger control-in with the psychological health. People who have received much social support have shown lower degrees of depression and other negative moods caused by physical illness (e.g. Brown, Nicassio & Wallston, 1989), so social support playing a significant role in inducing positive change in the life of chronically ill patients.

It is also evident from the literature that chronically ill patients use different coping strategies which help them in better and speedy recovery and with the use of active coping strategies produce more favorable outcomes such as less pain as well as depression, and better quality of life (Holmes & Stevenson, 1990). Use of positive coping is positively associated with the good quality of life (Holubova et al., 2018). Coping strategies (Active-focused, Active-distracting) were acting as a moderator in the relationship of state anger with environmental mastery and personal growth. Avoidance focused coping strategies and Active focused coping strategies were acting as a moderator for the relationship of state anger with psychological functioning, social relationships and environment. Active distracting coping strategies were acting as a moderator in the relationship of state anger with social relationships and environment. Active focused coping strategies were acting as a moderator for the relationship of anger control-In with Self-Acceptance, positive relations with others and autonomy. Avoidance focused coping strategies were acting as a moderator in the relationship of anger control-In with positive relations with others and autonomy.

Religious focused coping strategies were playing the role of a moderator in the relationship of anger control-In with positive relations with others and autonomy. Active focused coping strategies, Avoidance focused coping strategies and Avoidance focused coping strategies were acted as a moderator in the relationship of anger control-In with Physical functioning, Psychological functioning, Social relationships and Environment. Religious focused coping strategies were acted as a moderator in the relationship of anger control-In with Social relationships and Environment. Literature highlighted that the positive religious coping (positive thinking about God and positive beliefs related to him) have positive association with better quality of life, whereas the negative religious coping (anger with and on God) is negatively linked with the quality of life of the patients (Tarakeshwar, Vanderwerker, Paulk, Pearce, Kasl, & Prigerson, 2006). Active focused coping strategies were acting as a moderator in the relationship of anger control-in with the environment. By using different coping strategies patients are having a prominent effect on their psychological well-being and quality of life.

Role of Demographic Variables

MANOVA was computed on the demographic variables which were further explored with the ANOVA analysis. Significant MANOVA (multivariate) main effect of education and marital status, education with age was computed and then univariate analyses of variance was done, which indicated significant differences in depression, informational support, social network support, environmental mastery, self-acceptance, autonomy, purpose in life and personal growth. Results of independent sample t-test indicated that tangible support, environmental mastery, positive relations with others and personal growth is significantly high among female patients as compared to males. Although literature indicates that no significant difference has been reported for depression of male and female chronically ill patients with respect to social support (Berard, VanDenKerkhof, Harrison, & Tranmer, 2012). In Pakistani society mostly females are doing multitasking, they are home makers and also deals with the social ties. As females are very expressive so even in chronic illness they share their problems with family members and get tangible support whereas males do not share a lot that's why they are not asking for help and support so they are not getting tangible support as females are getting. Environmental mastery is high among females which mean that they have the capacity to manage effectively with her life. They are trained to make and maintain relations. It's in the grooming and broughtup of females in Pakistani society that they always put a lot of efforts in maintaining relationships and have high level of patients and tolerance with them. This also helps them in their personal growth. They are groomed in a manner in which they compromise and accept everything, which eventually helps them to develop self-acceptance. In chronic illness by sharing their pain they are not much affected by the chronic illness.

Pakistani culture is collectivistic in which people are closely connected with one another. It's natural that people want to share and when they share their pain and problems with others they feel relieved. People having joint family system, share a lot with each other so they don't have high or sever depression in contrast to those with nuclear family system. Those who are from the joint family system they share a strong and close bonding with one another. Whenever the support is needed it is always available and that is a very prominent feature of collectivistic culture. They expect a lot from one another that's why in case of any emergency or illness they come more and closer with one another (Cheema, Kaira & Bhugra, 2010). Present study results also revealed that depression is significantly high among those patients who are from nuclear family system whereas environmental mastery, positive relations with others and personal growth is high among those patients having joint family system. In joint family system because of lots of sharing and connectivity patients develop positive relations with others and it helps in their personal growth. With the help of family support and help patients can easily achieve environmental mastery.

Present study revealed that the depression and anger are commonly reported psychological issues among chronically ill patients (cancer, cardiac and diabetic patients). The coping strategies and social support play a role of risk and protective factor in their impact on quality of life and psychological well-being. They act as a moderator in relationship of psychological issues (depression and anger) with psychological well-being and quality of life, so there is a need to device a proper treatment plan for them for their health improvements.

Conclusion

The present study found that depression and anger are most commonly reported psychological issues among chronically ill patients. It also get highlighted that there is a significant negative relationship of depression and anger with quality of life (psychological functioning, physical functioning, environment and social relationship) and psychological well-being (autonomy, personal growth, positive relations with others, environmental mastery, self-acceptance and purpose in life) of the patients. Social support (tangible support, social network support) was explored as moderator in relationship between depression and psychological well- being (self - acceptance, positive relationship with other and autonomy), whereas esteem support acted as moderator between relationship of state anger and psychological well -being (environmental mastery, personal growth). The significant multivariate main effect of education and marital status, education with age, then univariate analyses of variance was computed, indicated the significant differences in depression, informational support, social network support, environmental mastery, self-acceptance, autonomy, purpose in life and personal growth. Tangible support, environmental mastery, positive relations with others and personal growth is significantly high among females patients as compared to males. Depression is significantly high among those patients who are from nuclear family system whereas environmental mastery, positive relations with others and personal growth is high among those patients having joint family system.

Implications

Present study assumes to have both implications, theoretical and practical. With reference to theoretical implications, the data collected through multi-informant approach to identify the psychological issues, risk and protective factors of patients (chronically ill), it is adding to the existing body of knowledge about this issue. Previously the data was collected from either patients or caregivers or doctors or nurses but in the present research multi-informant approach was used to have a clearer and broader understanding of the phenomenon. Multi-informant approach was used to get information from every possible source.

Secondly present study provides an indigenous scale for the assessment of anger. Although there are numerous scales on it but those are either covering the behavioral or the physical aspect or some of the instruments are for healthy individuals but this scale is for chronically ill patients and was developed by taking the mental condition of the chronically ill patients into consideration. It's in an Urdu language and easily understandable for the Pakistani population.

On practical grounds, it has its implication in clinical settings in devising a proper treatment plan which not only consider the bodily symptoms but also the psychological ones. Sometimes psychological issues are just signs and symptoms but if the attention is not paid then these signs and symptoms turn into syndrome, so attention is required in this regard. This study provides detailed rich information about the psychological issues, risk and protective factors, which can be used in educating the concerned caregivers, doctors and nurses about condition of patients.

Limitations and Future Suggestions

Along with the implications, present study also holds limitations. First of all the study was cross-sectional study so there is a need to conduct a longitudinal study to check out the psychological condition of the patients during the course of treatment. Longitudinal research design is important for clear casual inferences

Another limitation is that in present study only three chronic illnesses were taken, in future the more illnesses should be taken to check out the psychological issues, risk and protective factors with reference to well-being and quality of life of patients. Another limitation is that patients were taken from one hospital of Islamabad, in future data from other hospitals should be taken for comparison purpose. In present study sample was not very large, in future more nationally representative sample for the generalization purpose. As most of the patients were females so may be differneces among male and females are not very obvious so in future equivalent sample can be taken for more clear picture and for generalization of results. Future researches about should be conducted about the management and control of certain variables which may affect the well-being and quality of life of patients.

REFERENCES

Aaronson, N. K., Ahmedzai, S., Bergman, B., Bullinger, M., Cull, A., Duez, N. J.,...Kaasa, S. (1993). The European Organization for Research and Treatment of Cancer QLQ-C30: A quality-of-life instrument for use in international clinical trials in oncology. *JNCI: Journal of the National Cancer Institute, 85*(5), 365-376.

Abolfathi Momtaz, Y., Hamid, T. A., Ibrahim, R., Yahaya, N., & Abdullah, S. S. (2012). Moderating effect of Islamic religiosity on the relationship between chronic medical conditions and psychological well-being among elderly Malays. *Psychogeriatrics, 12*(1), 43-53.

Abraham, H. D., Degli-Esposti, S., & Marino, L. (1999). Seroprevalence of hepatitis C in a sample of middle class substance abusers. *Journal of Addictive Diseases, 18*(4), 77-87.

Abu-Helalah, M., Al-Hanaqta, M., Alshraideh, H., Abdulbaqi, N., & Hijazeen, J. (2014). Quality of life and psychological well-being of breast cancer survivors in Jordan. *Asian Pac J Cancer Prev, 15*(14), 5927-36.

Ali, I. (2018). The Nexus between CSR, corporate image, company identification, emotional attachment and small investors behavior. *Corporate Social Responsibility: Concepts, Methodologies, Tools, and Applications: Concepts, Methodologies, Tools, and Applications Critical explorations.* Management Association, Information Resources. IGI Global.

Alter, M. J., Kruszon-Moran, D., Nainan, O. V., McQuillan, G. M., Gao, F., Moyer, L. A.,...Margolis, H. S. (1999). The prevalence of hepatitis C virus infection in the United States, 1988 through 1994. *N Engl J Med., 34*, 556-562.

American Diabetes Association [ADA]. (2013). *Diabetes basics: Type 2.* Retrieved from http://www.diabetes.org/diabetes-basics/type-2/

Anderson, G., & Arsenault, N. (2005). *Fundamentals of educational research.* Canada: Arsenault-McGill

Anderson, R. J., Freedland, K. E., Clouse, R. E., & Lustman, P. J. (2001). The prevalence of co-morbid depression in adults with diabetes. *Diabetes Care, 24*, 1069–1078.

Ansari, S. A., (2010). Cross validation of Ryff scales of psychological well-being: Translation to Urdu language. *Pakistan Business Review, 12*(2), 244-259.

Asghsremoghadam, M. (2006). The role of associate beliefs with pain in adaptability with cancer. *Shahed University Research and Science Journal, 13*, 1-22.

Aziz, S., Noorulain, W., Zaidi, U. R., Hossain, K., & Siddiqui, I. A. (2009). Prevalence of overweight and obesity among children and adolescents of affluent schools in Karachi. *Journal of Pakistan Medical Association, 59*, 35-38.

Bailey, R. K., Geyen, D. J., Scott-Gurnell, K., Hipolito, M. M. S., Bailey, T. A., & Beal, J. M. (2005). Understanding and treating depression among cancer patients. *International Journal of Gynecologic Cancer, 15*(2), 203-208.

Bal, D. G., & Foerster, S. B. (1991). Changing the American diet: Impact on cancer prevention policy recommendations and program implications for the American Cancer Society. *Cancer, 67*(10), 2671-2680.

Ballesteros de Valderrama, B. P., Botero, C., Caycedo, C., Gutiérrez, M., Hermida, G., Medina, A., Montaña, P., Otero, M. (2003). *Revisión del concepto de Bienestar Psicológico.* Facultad de Psicología. Pontifcia Universidad Javeriana, Documento inédito

Ballesteros, B., & Caycedo, C. (2002). *El bienestar psicológico en el marco del análisis del comportamiento.* Facultad de Psicología. Pontifcia Universidad Javierana, Documento inédito.

Bano, S., Farhat, S. M., Arif, S., Mustaq, M., Zafar, M., Khurshid, F.,…Abro, M. M. (2013). *Report on awareness about cancer in Pakistan. National academy of young scientists school of biological sciences*. Lahore: University of Punjab.

Barefoot, J. C., & Schroll, M. (1996). Symptoms of depression, acute myocardial infarction, and total mortality in a community sample. *Circulation, 93*, 1976–1980.

Beck, A. T., Steer, R. A., & Carbin, M. G. (1988). Psychometric properties of the Beck Depression Inventory: Twenty-five years of evaluation. *Clinical psychology review, 8*(1), 77-100.

Belgrave, F. Z. (1998). *Psychosocial aspects of chronic illness and disability among African Americans*. USA: Greenwood.

Benjamin, E, J., Blaha, M, J., Chiuve, S., Cushman, M., Das, S. R., Deo, R.,...Muntner, P. (2017). Heart disease and stroke statistics – 2017 Update: A report from the American Heart Association. *Circulation, 135*, e146-e603.

Berard, D. M., VanDenKerkhof, E. G., Harrison, M., & Tranmer, J. E. (2012). Gender differences in the influence of social support on one-year changes in functional status in older patients with heart failure. *Cardiology Research and Practice, 2012*.

Berelson, B. (1952). *Content analysis in communication research*. Glencoe, IL: The Free Press.

Biondi, M., Picardi, A., Pasquini, M., Gaetano, P., & Pancheri, P. (2005). Dimensional psychopathology of depression: detection of an "activation" dimension in unipolar depressed oupatients. *Journal of Affective Disorders, 84*, 133–139. doi: 10.1016/S0165-0327(02)00103-9.

Bodurka-Bevers, D., Basen-Engquist, K., Carmack, C. L., Fitzgerald, M. A., Wolf, J. K., Moor, C. D., & Gershenson, D. M. (2000). Depression, anxiety, and quality of life in patient s with epthelial ovarian cancer. *Gynecologic Oncology, 78*, 302–308.

Boehm, J. K, Peterson, C., Kivimaki, M., & Kubzansky, L. (2011). A prospective study of positive psychological well-being and coronary heart disease. *Health Psychology, 30* (3), 259 – 267.

Bornbaum, C. C., Fung, K., Franklin, J. H., Nichols, A., Yoo, J., & Doyle, P. C. (2012). A descriptive analysis of the relationship between quality of life and distress in individuals with head and neck cancer. *Supportive Care in Cancer, 20*, 2157–2165.

Brannon, L., & Feist, J. (2009). *Health psychology: An introduction to behavior and health* (7th Ed.). USA: Cengage Learning.

Britneff, E., & Winkley, K. (2013). The role of psychological interventions for people with diabetes and mental health issues. *Journal of Diabetes Nursing, 17*(8), 305 – 310.

Brown, G. K., Nicassio, P. M., & Wallston, K. A. (1989). Pain coping strategies and depression in rheumatoid arthritis. *Journal of Consulting and Clinical Psychology, 57*(5), 652.

Brown, J. D. (2009). Principal components analysis and exploratory factor analysis &ndash Definitions, differences, and choices. *Statistics, 13*(1), 26-30.

Brown, R.T. (1999). *Cognitive aspects of chronic illness in children.* Guilford: Guilford Press.

Bryant, F. B., & Marquez, J. T. (1986). Educational status and the structure of subjective well-being m men and women. *Social Psychology Quarterly, 49*, 142-153.

Burish, T. G., & Bradley, L. A. (1983). *Coping with chronic disease: Research and applications.* New York: Academic Press.

Carney, R. M., & Freedland, K. E. (2008). Depression in patients with coronary heart disease. *The American journal of Medicine, 121*(11 supplement 2), 20-27. doi: 10.1016/j.amjmed.2008.09.010.

Carpio, C., Pacheco, V., Flores, C., & Canales, C. (2000). Calidad de Vida: un análisis de su dimensión psicológica. *Revista Sonorense de Psicología, 14*, 3-15.

Carver, C., & Abrahamson, M. (2009). Diabetes Mellitus overview. In K. Weinger & C. Carver (Eds), *Educating your patients with diabetes* (pp, 15-27). Boston: Humana Press.

Casper, D. R. (2015). *Predicting reasons for living among chronically ill and depressed middle aged and older adults enrolled in a randomized clinical trial.* Retrieved from https://ir.uiowa.edu/cgi/viewcontent.cgi?article=6294&context=etd

Cassileth, B. R., Lusk, E. J., Strouse, T. B., Miller, D.S., Brown, L.L., Cross, P. A.,…Tenaglia, A. N. (1984). Psychosocial status in chronic illness: A comparative analysis of six diagnostic groups. *New England Journal of Medicine, 311*, 506-511.

Castera, L., Constant, A., Bernard, P. H., Ledinghen, V. L., & Couzigor, P. (2006). Psychological impact of chronic hepatitis C: Comparison with other stressful events and chronic diseases. *World J Gastroenterology, 12*(10), 1545-1550.

Centers for Disease Control and Prevention [CDC]. (2007). *National diabetes fact sheet*. Retrieved from http://www.cdc.gov/diabetes/pubs/factsheet.htm.

Centers for Disease Control and Prevention [CDC]. (2013). *Death and mortality*. Retrieved from http://www.cdc.gov/nchs/fastats/deaths.htm.

Cheema, F., Kalra, G., & Bhugra, D. (2010). Globalisation and Mental Health: Context and Controversies. *Journal of Pakistan psychiatric society (JPPS)*, 7(2), 55-62.

Chen, H. Y., Baumgardner, D. J., & Rice, J. P. (2011). Peer reviewed: Health-related quality of life among adults with multiple chronic conditions in the United States, behavioral risk factor surveillance system, 2007. *Preventing Chronic Disease, 8*(1), A09.

Christensen, T., & Lægreid, P. (Eds.). (2002). *New public management: the transformation of ideas and practice*. Ashgate Pub Limited.

Cohen, S., & Rodriquez, M. S. (1995). Pathways linking affective disturbances and physical disorders. *Health Psychology, 14*, 374–380.

Compare, A., Zarbo, C., Manzoni, G. M., Castelnuovo, G., Baldassari, E., Bonardi, A., ... & Romagnoni, C. (2013). Social support, depression, and heart disease: a ten year literature review. *Frontiers in psychology*, 4, 384.

Crane, R.S. (1981). The role of anger, hostility and aggression in essential hyper tension. (Unpublished Doctoral Dissertation). University of South Florida. *Dissertation Abstracts International, 42*, 2982-B.

Crawford, J., Cayley, C., Lovibond, P. F., Wilson, P. H., & Hartley, C. (2011). Percentile norms and accompanying interval estimates from an Australian general adult population sample for self-report mood scales (BAI, BDI, CRSD, CES-D, DASS, DASS-21, STAI-X, STAI-Y, SRDS, and SRAS). *Australian Psychologist, 46*(1), 3-14.

Dahlen, E. R., & Deffenbacher, J. L. (2001). Anger management. In W. J. Lyddon & J. V. Jones (Eds.), *Empirically-supported cognitive therapies: Current status and future promise* (pp. 163-181). New York: Springer.

Dalal, A. K. (2015). *Health beliefs and coping with chronic diseases.* SAGE Publishing India.

Davidson, K. W., & Mostofsky, E. (2010). Anger expression and risk of coronary heart disease: evidence from the Nova Scotia Health Survey. *American Heart Journal, 159*(2), 199-206.

Dawood, S., & Yousaf, H. (2015). Spiritual Well-Being and Coping Styles in relation to Psychological Well-being of Adolescents. *Pakistan Journal of Social and Clinical Psychology, 13*(2), 48-52.

Deci, E., & Ryan, R. (Eds.). (2002). *Handbook of self-determination research.* Rochester, NY: University of Rochester Press.

Derogatis, L, R., Morrow, G, R., & Fetting, J., Penman, D., Piasetsky, S., Schmale, A. M.,…Carnicke, C. L. (1983). The prevalence of psychiatric disorders among cancer patients. *JAMA, 249,* 751–757.

Diabetics Institute Pakistan [DIP]. (2013). *Diabetes statistics in Pakistan.* Retrieved from http://diabetespakistan.com/treatement/ABC-of-Diabetes/2013/10/05/diabetes-sttaistics-in-pakistan/

Diener, E. (2009). Subjective well-being. *The Science of Well-Being,* 11-58.

Diener, E. D., Oishi, S., & Lucas, R. E. (2003). Personality, culture and subjective well-being: Emotional and cognitive evaluations of life. *Annaul Review of Psychology, 54,* 403-425. Retrieved from http://www.findarticles.com/p/articles/mi-s42587/is-n127-v56/ai-1094145605.pg-3

DiGiuseppe, R., & Tafrate, R. C. (2007). *Understanding anger disorders.* Oxford University Press.

Dubey, A. (2012). *Psychological perspectives on chronic illnesses.* India: Concept Publishing.

Edward, K. L. (2013). Chronic illness and wellbeing: using nursing practice to foster resilience as resistance. *British Journal of Nursing, 22*(13), 741-746.

Etzler, S. L, Rohrmann, S., & Brandt, H. (2014). Validation of the STAXI-2: A study with prison inmates. *Psychological Test and Assessment Modeling, 56*(2), 178-194.

Falvo, D. R. (2005). *Medical and psychosocial aspects of chronic illness and disability* (3rd ed.). USA: Jones & Bartlett.

Falvo, D., & Holland, B. E. (2017). *Medical and psychosocial aspects of chronic illness and disability.* Jones & Bartlett Learning.

Felitti, V. J., Anda, R. F., Nordenberg, D., Williamson, D. F., Spitz, A. M., Edwards, V.,...Marks, J. S. (1998). Relationship of childhood abuse and household dysfunction to many of the leading causes of death in adults: The Adverse Childhood Experiences (ACE) Study. *American Journal of Preventive Medicine, 14*(4), 245-258.

Ferrando, P. J., & Lorenzo-Seva U. (2016). A note on improving EAP trait estimation in oblique factor-analytic and item response theory models. *Psicologica, 37,* 235-247.

Ferrell, B. (1995). The impact of pain on quality of life: A decade of research. *The Nursing Clinics of North America, 30*(4), 609.

Field, A. (2005). *Discovering statistics using SPSS* (2nd ed.). London: Sage.

Frank-Stromborg, M., & Olsen, S. (2004). *Instruments for clinical health-care research.* Jones & Bartlett Learning.

Fredrikson-Golden, K. I. (2007). HIV/AIDS care giving: Predictors of wellbeing and distress. *Journal of Gay and Lesbian Social Services, 18,* 53 – 73.

Friedman, S. (2000). Cardiac disease, anxiety and sexual functioning. *American Journal of Cardiology, 86,* 46F–50F.

Garavito, L. (2001). *Calidad de vida y toma de decisiones médicas* (Unpublished Doctoral dissertation). Tesis de especialidad en bioética. Pontificia Universidad Javeriana. Documento Inédito.

George, D., & Mallery, M. (2010). *Using SPSS for Windows step by step: A simple guide and reference.* Boston, MA: Allyn & Bacon.

Ghazanfar, L., & Shafiq, S. (2016). Coping strategies and family functioning as predictors of stress among caregivers of mentally ill patients. *International Journal of Clinical Psychiatry, 4*, 8-16.

Ghosh, S. (2015). Inflammatory bowel disease: appreciating disability and impact of disease. *Canadian Journal of Gastroenterology and Hepatology, 29*(2), 66-66.

Goepp, C., & Hammond, W. (1977). *Terapia de Apoyo del Paciente Canceroso*. Buenos Aires: Médica Panamericana.

Gómez, M. M. N., Gutiérrez, R. M. V., Castellanos, S. A. O., Vergara, M. P., & Pradilla, Y. K. R. (2010). Psychological well-being and quality of life in patients treated for thyroid cancer after surgery. *Terapia psicológica, 28*(1), 69-84.

Gómez, M. M. N., Gutiérrez, R. M. V., Castellanos, S. A. O., Vergara, M. P., & Pradilla, Y. K. R. (2010). Psychological well-being and quality of life in patients treated for thyroid cancer after surgery. *Terapia psicológica, 28*(1), 69-84.

Grau, J., & Pörtero, D (1987). *Perspectivas del Estudio del Cuadro Interno de las Enfermedades*. En Memorias del Congreso Colombiano de Psicología Clínica. acultad de Psicología de la undación Universitaria de Manizales, Colombia.

Greenberg, T. (2007). *The psychological impact of acute and chronic illness: A practical guide for primary care physicians*. San Francisco: Springer Science & Business Media.

Gregurek, R., Braš, M., Đor đ ević, V., Ratkovi ć, A., & Brajković, L., (2010). Psychological problems of patients with cancer. *Psychiatria Danubina, 22*(2), 227-230.

Guthrie, E. (1996). Emotional disorder in chronic illness: psychotherapeutic interventions. *British Journal Psychiatry, 168*(3), 265-73.

Hadi, N., Asadollahi, R., & Talei, A. R. (2009). Anxiety, depression and anger in breast cancer patients compared with the general population in Shiraz, Southern Iran. *Iranian Red Crescent Medical Journal, 11*(3), 312-317.

Harris, C. A., & Joyce, L. D. (2008). Psychometric properties of the Beck Depression Inventory-(BDI-II) in individuals with chronic pain. *PAIN®, 137*(3), 609-622.

Hayes, A. F., & Krippendorff, K. (2007). Answering the call for a standard reliability measure for coding data. *Communication Methods and Measures, 1*, 77-89.

Heather, S. J., Susan, A. R., Deanna, M. G., & Barbara, L. A. (2006). Strategies used in coping with a cancer diagnosis predict meaning in life for survivors. *Health Psychology, 25*(6), 753–761.

Helgeson, V. S., & Cohen, S. (1996). Social support and adjustment to cancer: reconciling descriptive, correlational, and intervention research. *Health Psychology, 15*(2), 135.

Heller, N. R., & Gitterman, A. (2010). *Mental health and social problems: A social work perspective.* USA: Taylor & Francis.

Hermanns, N., Kulzer, B., Krichbaum, M., Kubiak, T., & Haak, T. (2006) How to screen for depression and emotional problems in patients with diabetes: comparison of screening characteristics of depression questionnaires, measurement of diabetes-specific emotional problems and standard clinical assessment. *Diabetologia, 49*, 469-477.

Hisham, R., Ng, C. J., Liew, S. M., Lai, P. S. M., Chia, Y. C., Khoo, E. M., ... & Chinna, K. (2018). Development and validation of the Evidence Based Medicine Questionnaire (EBMQ) to assess doctors' knowledge, practice and barriers regarding the implementation of evidence-based medicine in primary care. *BMC family practice, 19*(1), 98.

Holländare, F., Andersson, G., & Engström, I. (2010). A comparison of psychometric properties between internet and paper versions of two depression instruments (BDI-II and MADRS-S) administered to clinic patients. *Journal of medical Internet research, 12*(5), e49.

Holmes, J. A., & Stevenson, C. A. (1990). Differential effects of avoidant and attentional coping strategies on adaptation to chronic and recent-onset pain. *Health Psychology, 9*(5), 577.

Holubova, M., Prasko, J., Ociskova, M., Grambal, A., Slepecky, M., Marackova, M., ... & Zatkova, M. (2018). Quality of life and coping strategies of outpatients with a depressive disorder in maintenance therapy–a cross-sectional study. *Neuropsychiatric Disease and Treatment, 14*, 73.

Honorato, N. P., Abumusse, L. V. D. M., Coqueiro, D. P., & Citero, V. D. A. (2017). Personality traits, anger and psychiatric symptoms related to quality of life in patients with newly diagnosed digestive system cancer. *Arquivos de Gastroenterologia, 54*(2), 156-162.

Hosoda, S., Takimura, H., Shibayama, M., Kanamura, H., Kenji, I., & Kumada, H. (2000). Psychiatric symptoms related to interferon therapy for chronic hepatitis C: Clinical features and prognosis. *Psychiatry and Clinical Neurosciences, 54* (5), 565–572. Retrieved from http://www.blackwell-synergy.com/links/doi/10.1046/j.1440-1819.2000.00754.x

Huang, C. Y., & Hsu, M. C. (2013). Social support as a moderator between depressive symptoms and quality of life outcomes of breast cancer survivors. *European Journal of Oncology Nursing, 17*(6), 767-774.

Huang, M. F. (2009). *Resilience in chronic disease: The relationships among risk factors, protective factors, adaptive outcomes, and the level of resilience in adults with diabetes* (Doctoral dissertation, Queensland University of Technology).

Huffman, J. C., Legler, S. R., & Boehm, J. K. (2017). Positive psychological well-being and health in patients with heart disease: A brief review. *Future Cardiology, 13*(5). doi: 10.2217/fca-2017-0016.

Ilić, I., Šipetić-Grujičić, S., Grujičić, J., Živanović Mačužić, I., Kocić, S., & Ilić, M. (2019). Psychometric properties of the world health organization's quality of life (WHOQOL-BREF) questionnaire in medical students. *Medicina, 55*(12), 772.

Ilić, S., & Apostolovic, S. (2002). Psychological aspects of cardiovascular diseases. *Medicine and Biology, 9*(2), 138-141.

Ingram, R. E., & Luxton, D. D. (2005). Vulnerability–stress models. In B. L. Hankin & J. R. Z. Abela (Eds.), *Development of psychopathology: A vulnerability–stress perspective*. Thousand Oaks CA: Sage Publications.

Jafar, T. H., Haaland, B. A., Rahman, A., Razzak, J. A., Bilger, M., Naghavi, M.,…Hyder, A.A. (2013). Non-communicable diseases and injuries in

Pakistan: strategic priorities. *Lancet, 381,* 2281-2290. doi: 10.1016/S0140-6736(13)60646-7.

Javaid, A. (2014). Role of personality hardiness, self-efficacy, and social support in predicting resilience among health, hypertensive, and diabetic persons. Unpublished M.Phil Dissertation. National Institute of Psychology. Quaid-i-Azam University, Islamabad, Pakistan.

Jibeen, T., & Khalid, R. (2010). Predictors of psychological well-being of Pakistani immigrants in Toronto, Canada. *International Journal of intercultural relations, 34*(5), 452-464.

Jibeen, T., & Khalid, R. (2012). Cross Validation of Ryff's Scales of Psychological Well-being: Translation into Urdu Language Tahira Jibeen Department of Humanities COMSATS Institute of Information and Technology, Lahore, Pakistan. *International Journal, 10,* 2.

Kafka, G. J., & Kozma, A. (2002). The construct validity of Ryff's Scale of Psychological Well-Being (SPWB) and their relationship to measures of subjective well-being. *Social Indicators Research, 57*(2), 171-190.

Kasl, S. V., Chishoim, R. F., & Eskenazi, B. (1981). The impact of the Tree Mile Islands on the behavior and well-being of nuclear workers. *American Journal of Public Health, 71,* 484-495.

Katon, W. J. (2011). Epidemiology and treatment of depression in patients with chronic medical illness. *Dialogues in Clinical Neuroscience, 13*(1), 7.

Katon, W., & Sullivan, M. (1990). Depression and chronic medical illness. *Journal of Clinical Psychiatry, 51*(suppl 6), 3–11.

Kausar, R., & Munir, R. (2004). Pakistani adolescents' coping with stress: effects of loss of a parent and gender of adolescents. *Journal of Adolescence, 27,* 599-610.

Kausar, R., & Yusuf, S. (2011). State anxiety and coping strategies used by patients with hepatitis C in relation to interferon therapy. *Pakistan Journal of Social and Clinical Psychology, 9*(1), 57-61.

Keyes, C. L. M., & Lopez, S. J. (2002). Toward a science of mental health. In C. R. Snyder, & S. J. Lopez (Eds.), *Handbook of positive psychology* (pp. 45-59). Oxford: Oxford University Press.

Khan, A. A., Marwat, S. K., Noor, M. M., & Fatima, S. (2015). Reliability and validity of Beck Depression Inventory among general population in Khyber Pakhtunkhwa, Pakistan. *Journal of Ayub Medical College Abbottabad, 27*(3), 573-575.

Khan, J. (1996). *Validation and Norm Development of Salma Shah Depression Scale (SSDS)* (Unpublished M.Sc Research Report). Department of Psychology. University of Peshawar, Peshawar, Pakistan.

Kim, E., Han, J. Y., Shah, D., Shaw, B., McTavish, F., Gustafson, D. H.,…Fan, D. (2011). Predictors of supportive message expression and reception in an interactive cancer communication system. *Journal of Health Communication, 16*(10), 1106-1121. doi: 10.1080/10810730.2011.571337.

Kline, P. (1993). *Personality: The psychometric view.* London: Rutledge.

Koenig, H. G, Cohen, H. J, Blazer, D. G, Pieper, C, Meador, K. G, & Shelp F.,…DePasquale, B. (1992). Religious coping and depression among elderly, hospitalized medically ill men. *Am J Psychiatry, 149*, 1693-700. doi: 10.1176/ajp.149.12.1693.

Koot, M. H., & Wallender, J. L. (2001). *Quality of life in child and adolescent illness: Concepts, methods and findings.* Sussex: Brunner-Routledge.

Kraus, M. R., Schafer, A., Faller, H., Csef, H., & Scheurlen, M. (2004). *Psychiatric symptoms in patients with chronic hepatitis C receiving interferon alfa-2b therapy.* Retrieved from http://www.ncbi.nlm.nih.gov/entrez/query.

Kugaya, A., Akechi, T., Okuya ma, T., Nakano, T., Mikami, I., Okamura, H.,…Uchitomi, Y. (2000). Prevalence, predictive factors, and screening for psychological distress in patients with newly diagnosed head and neck cancer. *Cancer, 88*, 2817–2823.

Kühner, C., Bürger, C., Keller, F. and Hautzinger, M. (2007) Reliability and Validity of the Revised Beck Depression Inventory (BDI-II). Results from German

Samples. *Der Nervenarzt, 78*, 651-656. http://dx.doi.org/10.1007/s00115-006-2098-7

Lewko, J., & Misiak, B. (2015). Relationships between Quality of Life, Anxiety, Depression and Diabetes. *Annals of Depression and Anxiety, 2*(1), 10-40.

Lichtenstein, P., Holm, N. V., Verkasalo, P. K., Iliadou, A., Kaprio, J., Koskenvuo, M., ... & Hemminki, K. (2000). Environmental and heritable factors in the causation of cancer—analyses of cohorts of twins from Sweden, Denmark, and Finland. *New England journal of medicine, 343*(2), 78-85.

Lodhi, F. S., Raza, O., Montazeri, A., Nedjat, S., Yaseri, M., & Holakouie-Naieni, K. (2017). Psychometric properties of the Urdu version of the World Health Organization's quality of life questionnaire (WHOQOL-BREF). *Medical journal of the Islamic Republic of Iran, 31*, 129.

López, M., & Torres, G. (2001). *Estudios sobre calidad de vida en pacientes con cáncer en tratamiento de quimioterapia.* Tesis de maestría, Pontificia Universidad Javeriana.

Lubkin, I. M., & Larsen, P. D. (2006). *Chronic illness: Impact and interventions* (6th ed.). USA: Jones & Bartlett.

Lubkin, I. M., & Larsen, P. D. (2013). *Chronic illness: Impact and prevention* (8th ed.). USA: Jones & Bartlett.

Lustman, P. J., Clouse, R. E., Griffith, L. S., Carney, R. M., & Freedland, K. E. (1997). Screening for depression in diabetes using the Beck Depression Inventory. *Psychosomatic Medicine, 59*, 24–31.

Malik, A. M. (2002). *The study of social support as a determining factor in depressed and nondepressed as measured by an indigenously development Social Support Scale.* Karachi: Department of Psychology, University of Karachi.

Manzoor, Y. (2009). Relationship between social support and psychological wellbeing among incarcerated juveniles. (Unpublished M.Sc Dissertation), National Institute of Psychology, Quaid - i - Azam University, Islamabad, Pakistan.

Mir, K., Mir, K., Malik, I., & Shehzadi, A. (2015). Prevalence of co-morbid depression in diabetic population. *Journal of Ayub Medical College Abbottabad, 27*(1), 99-101.

Mitnick, S., Leffler, C., & Hood, V.L. (2009). Family caregivers, patients and physicians: Ethical guidance to optimize relationships. *Journal of General Internal Medicine, 25*(3), 255-256. doi: 10.1007/s11606-009-1206-3.

Mohamed, R., Abdul Kadir, A., & Yaacob, L. H. (2012). A study on depression among patient with type 2 diabetes mellitus in North-Eastcoast Malaysia. *International Journal of Collaborative Research on Internal Medicine & Public Health, 4*(8), 1589-600.

Murray, C. (2003). Risk factors, protective factors, vulnerability, and resilience: A framework for understanding and supporting the adult transitions of youth with high-incidence disabilities. *Remedial and Special Education, 24*(1), 16-26.

Muscatello, M. R., Troili, G. M., Pandolfo, G., Mento, C., Gallo, G., Lanza, G.,...Bruno, A. (2017). Depression, anxiety and anger in patients with type 1 diabetes mellitus. *Recenti Progressi in Medicina, 108*(2), 77-82.

Mushtaq, M., & Zubair, A. (2015).Group differences in functional impairment, social support and academic achievement among adolescents. *FWU Journal of Social Sciences, 9*(1), 33-43.

Muthén, B., & Kaplan, D. (1985). A comparison of some methodologies for the factor analysis of non-normal Likert variables. *British Journal of Mathematical and Statistical Psychology, 38*(2), 171-189.

National Cancer Registry (NCR) Malaysia. (2003). *Second Report of the National Cancer Registry, Cancer Incidence in Malaysia.* Kuala Lumpur, Malaysia: National Cancer Registry. Retrieved from http://www.care.upm.edu.my /dokumen/13603_2ndNCR2003.pdf.

Naveed, A., & Yousaf, A. (2015). Personality traits, coping startegies and social support in patients with depression and anxiety. *International Journal of scientific research and management. 3* (5), 2854 - 2865

Negovan, V. (2010). Dimensions of students' psychosocial well-being and their measurement: Validation of a students' Psychosocial Well Being Inventory. *Europe's Journal of Psychology, 6*(2), 85-104.

Newacheck, P. W., Strickland, B., Shonkoff, J. P., Perrin, J. M., Mc Pherson, M., McManus, M.,…Arango, P. (1998). An epidemiological profile of children with special health care needs. *Pediatrics, 102*(1), 117-123.

Newton, C. (2013). *Understanding mental disorder.* Retrieved from http://www.clairenewton.co.za/understanding-mental-disorders.html#h5-diathesis-stress-model.

Novoa, M. (2004) Pertinencia de las interacciones entre la ciencia médica yla psicología. In G. L. Oblitas (Ed.), *Manual de la psicología clínicay de la salud hospitalaria.* Retrieved from www.psicologiacientica.com.

Novoa, M. M., Cruz W, C., Rojas, S. L., y & Wilde, W. K. (2003). Efectos secundarios de los tratamientos de cáncer de prostate localizado, calidad de vida y ajuste marital. *Universitas Psychologica, 2,*169-186.

Novoa-Gómez, M. M., & Ballesteros, B. P. (2006). The role of the psychologist in an intensive care unit. *Universitas Psychologica,* 5, 599-613.

Novoa-Gómez, M. M., Moreno, I. S., Garcia, M. P., Leguizamón, L., & Castaño, I. (2006). Asociación entre el síndrome de estrés asistencial en residentes de medicina interna el reporte de sus prácticas subóptimas y el reporte de los pacientes. *Universitas Psychologica, 5,* 549-563.

Nunnally, J. C., & Bernstein, I. H. (1994). *Psychological theory.* New York, NY: MacGraw-Hill.

NVSS. (2013). Deaths: Final data for 2010. *National Vital Statistics Report, 61* (4), 1-117.

Ogden, J. (2012). *Health Psychology: A Textbook: A textbook.* McGraw-Hill Education (UK).

Oh, D. H., Kim, S. A., Lee, H. Y., Seo, J. Y., Choi, B. Y., & Nam, J. H. (2013). Prevalence and correlates of depressive symptoms in Korean adults: Results of a 2009 Korean community health survey. *Journal of Korean medical science, 28*(1), 128-135.

Ohaeri, J. U., &Awadalla, A. W. (2009). The reliability and validity of the short version of the WHO Quality of life instrument in an Arab general population. *Annals of Saudi Medicine, 29*(2). 98-104.

Okun, M. A., & Stock, W. A. (1987). The construct validity of subjective well-being measures: An assessment via quantitative research syntheses. *Journal of Community Psychology, 15*(4), 481-492.

Pariante, C, Orru, M., Baita, A., Farsi, M. G., & Carpiniello, B. (1999). Treatment with interferon-alpha in patients with chronic hepatitis and mood or anxiety disorders. *Lancet, 354*, 131-132.

Pasquini, M., & Biondi, M. (2007). Depression in cancer patients: a critical review. *Clinical Practice & Epidemiology in Mental Health, 3*, 2. doi: 10.1186/1745-0179-3-2

Pasquini, M., Picardi, A., Biondi, M., Gaetano, P., & Morosini, P. (2004). Relevance of anger and irritability in outpatients with major depressive disorder. *Psychopathology, 37*, 155–160. doi: 10.1159/000079418.

Pattern, S. B. (2001). Long-term medical conditions and major depression in a Canadian population study at waves 1 and 2. *Journal of Affective Disorders, 63*(1-3), 35-41.

Penckofer, S., Ferrans, C. E., Velsor-Friedrich, B., & Savoy, S. (2007). The psychological impact of living with diabetes women's day-to-day experiences. *The Diabetes Educator, 33*(4), 680-690.

Pouwer, F, Beekman, A. T, Lubach, C., & Snoek, F. J. (2006). Nurses' recognition and registration of depression, anxiety and diabetes-specific emotional problems in outpatients with diabetes mellitus. *Patient EducCouns, 60*, 235-240.

Power, M., Harper, A., & Bullinger, M. (1999). The World Health Organization WHOQOL-100: Tests of the University of quality of life in 15 different cultural group worldwide. *Health Psychology, 18*, 495-505.

Que, J. C., Sy Ortin, T. T., Anderson, K. O., Gonzalez-Suarez, C. B., Feeley, T. W., & Reyes-Gibby, C. C. (2013). Depressive symptoms among cancer patients in a

Philippine tertiary hospital: prevalence, factors, and influence on health-related quality of life. *Journal of Palliative Medicine, 16*(10), 1280-1284.

Quek, K. F., Low, W. Y., Razack, A. H., & Loh, C. S. (2001). A Malaysian Study on the reliability and validity of the Health-Related Quality of Life Questionnaire (HRQOL-20) in urological patients. *The Medical journal of Malaysia, 56*(3), 293-301.

Rabkin, J. G., Reimen, R., Katoff, L., & Williams, J. B. (1993). Resilience in adversity among long-term survivors of AIDS. *Hosp Community Psychiatry, 44*(2), 162-167.

Ramkisson, S., Pillay, B. J., & Sartorius, B. (2016). Anxiety, depression and psychological well-being in a cohort of South African adults with Type 2 diabetes mellitus. *South African Journal of Psychiatry, 22*(1). Retrieved from https://sajp.org.za/index.php/sajp/article/view/935/662.

Rezia, R., Islam, A., & Islam, S. M. S. (2018). Depressive symptoms among participants with type 2 diabetes in Southeast Asia: A systematic review. *Journal of Diabetology, 9*(1), 19. doi: 10.4103/jod.jod_23_17.

Rodríguez-Marin, J. (1998). *Psicología social de la salud.* Madrid: Síntesis.

Ryff, C. D., & Keyes, C. L. M. (1995). The structure of psychological well-being revisit Ed. *Journal of Personality and Social Psychology, 69*, 719–727.

Schlosser, B. (1990). The assessment of subjective well-being and its relationship to the stress process. *Journal of Personality Assessment, 54*(1-2), 128-140.

Schneiderman, N., (2004). Psychosocial, behavioral, and biological aspects of chronic diseases. *America Psychological Society, 13*(6), 247-251.

Seligman, M. E. P. (2002). *Authentic happiness: Using the new positive psychology to realize your potential for lasting fulfillment.* New York: Free Press.

Senescus, R. A. (1963). The development of emotional complications in patients with cancer. *J Chronic Dis., 16*, 813–832.

Shahid, A., Wilkinson, K., Marcu, S., & Shapiro, C. M. (Eds.). (2012). *STOP, THAT and one hundred other sleep scales.* Springer Science & Business Media.

Shapiro, P. (1996). Psychiatric aspects of cardiovascular disease. *Psychiatric Clinics of North America, 19*, 613-628.

Sheldon, K. M., Ryan, R., & Reis, H. T. (1996). What makes for a good day? Competence and autonomy in the day and in the person. *Personality and Social Psychology Bulletin, 22*(12), 1270-1279.

Short, P. F., Vasey, J. J., & Belue, R. (2008). Work disability associated with cancer survivorship and other chronic conditions. *Psychooncology, 17,* 91-7.

Siegel, J. M. (1986). The Multidimensional Anger Inventory. *Journal of Personality and Social Psychology. 51*(1), 191-200. doi: 10.1037/0022-3514.51.1.191.

Sinha, J. N. P., & Verma, J. (1992). Social support as a moderator of the relationship between allocentrism and psychological well-being. In U. Kim, H.C. Triandis, Ç. Kâgitçibasi, S. Choi & G. Yoon (Eds.), *Individualism and collectivism* (pp. 267-275). Thousand Oaks, CA: Sage.

Snyder, I., & Lopez, J. (2002). Coping with adversity. *The International Journal of Social Psychology, 40*(2), 35-45.

Solowiejczyk, J. (2010). *Diabetes and depression: Some thoughts to think about.* American Diabetes Association: Diabetes Spectrum. Retrieved from http://spectrum.diabetesjournals.org/content/23/1/11.full-text.pdf.

Spiegel, D., & Kato, P. M., (1996). Psychosocial influences on cancer incidence and progression. *Harv Rev Psychiatry, 4,* 10-26.

Spielberger, C. D. (1988). *State-Trait-Anger-Expression-Inventory.* Palo Alto, CA: Consulting Psychologist Press.

Spielberger, C. D. (1999). Sta*te-Trait Anger Expression Inventory-2 (STAXI-2): Professional Manual.* Tampa, FL: Psychological Assessment Resources.

Šprah, L., & Šoštarič, M. (2004). Psychosocial coping strategies in cancer patients. *Radiology and Oncology, 38*(1), 35-42. Retrieved from https://www.radioloncol.com/index.php/ro/article/view/1349/1107.

Šprah, L., & Šoštarič, M. (2004). Psychosocial coping strategies in cancer patients. *Radiology and Oncology, 38*(1).

Streiner, D. L., Norman, G. R., & Cairney, J. (2015). *Health measurement scales: a practical guide to their development and use.* Oxford University Press, USA.

Swindells, S., Mohr, J., Justis, J. C., Berman, S., Squier, C., Wagener, M. M.,...Singh, N. (1999). Quality of life in patients with human immunodeficiency virus infection: impact of social support, coping style and hopelessness. *International journal of STD & AIDS, 10*(6), 383-391.

Tarakeshwar, N., Vanderwerker, L. C., Paulk, E., Pearce, M. J., Kasl, S. V., & Prigerson, H. G. (2006). Religious coping is associated with the quality of life of patients with advanced cancer. *Journal of palliative medicine, 9*(3), 646-657.

Taylor, D. R. (2009). *Abnormal glucose tolerance and insulin resistance in treated patients with essential hypertension* (Unpublished Master's thesis). University of Witwatersrand, Johannesburg. Retrieved from http://wiredspace.wits.ac.za/bitstream/handle/10539/12162/D_R_Taylor.pdf?sequence=1

Taylor, E. J., Baird, S. B., Malone, D., & McCorkle, R. (1993). Factors associated with anger in cancer patients and their caregivers. *Cancer practice, 1*(2), 101-109.

Taylor, S. E. (2006). *Health psychology*. India: Tata McGraw-Hill Education

Tuncay, T., Musabak, I., Gok, D. E., & Kutlu, M. (2008). The relationship between anxiety, coping strategies and characteristics of patients with diabetes. *Health Quality Life Outcomes, 6*, 79.

Turner, J., & Brian, K. (2000). Emotional dimensions of chronic disease. *The Western Journal of Medicine, 172*(2), 124-128.

Turner, S. (1995). Family variables related to adolescent substance misuse: Risk and resiliency factors. In T. R. Gullotto, G. R. Adams, & R. Montemayor (Eds.), *Substance misuse in adolescence*. Thousand Oaks, CA: Sage.

United Nations News Centre. (2012, May 16). *Hypertension and diabetes on the rise worldwide, says UN report.* Retrieved from http://www.un.org/apps/newsstory/.asp?NewsID=40950&Cr=non_communicable+disease&Cr1=

Van De Ven, M. O., Engels, R. C., Sawyer, S. M., Otten, R., & Van Den Eijnden, R. J. (2007). The role of coping strategies in quality of life of adolescents with asthma. *Quality of Life Research, 16*(4), 625-634.

Verhaak, P. F. M., Heijmans, M. J. W. M., Peters, & Rijken, M. (2005). Chronic disease and mental disorder. *Social Science & Medicine, 60*(4), 789-797.

Vila, G., Hayder, R., Bertrand, C., Falissard, B., De Blic, J., Mouren-Simeoni, M. C.,...Scheinmann, P. (2003). Psychopathology and quality of life for adolescents with asthma and their parents. *Psychosomatics, 44*(4), 319-28.

Vu, H. T. T., Nguyen, T. X., Nguyen, H. T. T., Le, T. A., Nguyen, T. N., Nguyen, A. T.,...Latkin, C. A. (2018). Depressive symptoms among elderly diabetic patients in Vietnam. *Diabetes, Metabolic Syndrome and Obesity: Targets and Therapy, 11,* 659.

Wagner, E. H., Austin, B. T., Davis, C., Hindmarsh, M., Schaefer, J., & Bonomi, A. (2014). Improving chronic illness care: Translating evidence into action. *Health Affairs, 20*(6), 64-78.

Wallander, J. L., & Varni, J. W. (1998). Effects of pediatric chronic physical disorder on child and family adjustment. *Journal of Child Psychology and Psychiatry, 39,* 29-46.

Ward, B. W., Schiller, J. S., & Goodman, R. A. (2014). Multiple chronic conditions among Us adults: A 2012 update. *Centers for Disease Control and Prevention, 11,* 130389. doi: http://dx.doi.org/10.5888/pcd11.130389.

Watson, D., Clark, L. A., & Tellengen, A. (1988). Development and validation of brief measures of positive and negative affect: the PANAS scales. *Journal of Personality and Social Psychology, 54,* 1063-1070.

Weihs, K. L., Enright, T. M., & Simmens, S. J. (2008). Close relationships and emotional processing predict decreased mortality in women with breast cancer: preliminary evidence. *Psychosomatic Medicine, 70*(1), 117-124.

Wells, K. B., Golding, J. M., & Burnam, M. A. (1988). Psychiatric disorder in a sample of the general population with and without chronic medical conditions. *American Journal of Psychiatry, 145,* 976–981.

WFMH. (2010). *Mental health and chronic physical illnesses: The need for continued and integrated care.* Retrieved from http://www.wfmh.org/2010DOCS/WMHDAY2010.pdf

WHO. (2005). *Preventing chronic diseases: A vital investment: WHO global report*. Geneva: World Health Organization.

WHO. (2011). *Media centre: Asthma*. Retrieved from http://www.who.int/mediacentre/factsheets/fs307/en/index.html

WHO. (2011). *Media centre: Cardiovascular disease (CVDs)*. Retrieved from http://www.who.int/mediacentre/factsheets/fs317/en/index.html

WHO. (2012). *World Health Organization: Chronic diseases*. Retrieved from http://www.who.int/topics/chronic_diseases/en/

WHO. (2013). *Non–Communicative diseases*. Retrieved from http://www.who.int/mediacentre/factsheets/fs355/en/

WHO. (2014). *World Health Organization – Noncommunicable Diseases (NCD) Country Profile*. Retrieved from www.who.int/nmh/countries/pak_en.pdf?ua=1.

WHO. (2017). *Cardiovascular diseases (CVDs)*. Retrieved from www.who.int/mediacentre/factsheets/fs317/en/.

World Health Organization. WHO. (2006). *Constitution of the World Health Organization – Basic Documents*, Forty-fifth edition, Supplement, October 2006.

Wu, S. F. V. (2014). Rapid screening of psychological well-being of patients with chronic illness: reliability and validity test on WHO-5 and PHQ-9 scales. *Depression Research and Treatment, 2014*, 239490. doi: 10.1155/2014/239490

Yusof, S., Zakaria, F. N., Hashim, N. K., & Dasiman, R. (2016). Depressive Symptoms among Cancer Patients Undergoing Chemotherapy. *Procedia-Social and Behavioral Sciences, 234*, 185-192.

Zebrack, B. J. (2011). Psychological, social, and behavioral issues for young adults with cancer. *Cancer, 117*(10 suppl), 2289–2294.